Ethics and Palli

A case-based manual

Edited by

Roger Worthington

With contributions from

Paddy Stone and Andrew Thorns

Foreword by

Teresa Tate

Radcliffe Publishing

Radcliffe Publishing Ltd
18 Marcham Road
Abingdon
Oxon OX14 1AA
United Kingdom

www.radcliffe-oxford.com
Electronic catalogue and worldwide online ordering facility.

British Library Cataloguing in Publication Data

A catalogue record for this book is available from the British Library.

ISBN 1 85775 846 3

Typeset by Action Publishing Technology Limited, Gloucester
Printed and bound by TJ International Ltd, Padstow, Cornwall

Contents

Foreword

'I come now to mention the moral qualities peculiarly required in the character of a physician. The chief of these is humanity; that sensibility of heart which makes us feel for the distress of our fellow creatures, and which, of consequence, incites us in the most powerful manner to relief them.'

John Gregory 1724–1773

Over the past few years the recognition that an ethical perspective should play a central part in clinical decision making has moved from the sidelines into the mainstream of practice. It is, however, apparent that many healthcare practitioners feel poorly informed about the principles of ethical thought and uncertain about how to apply them to their day-to-day practice. A sense that 'ethics' is a separate, different component of care, in some way divided from the main processes of medical treatment, still persists. Medical text books still contain discrete chapters on ethics which helps to reinforce this impression of displacement from the core of daily practice.

The ability to apply practical ethical thinking to clinical problems arises from an understanding of our own moral setting; of the events and influences which have shaped us and which we bring to bear on our practice and on our interactions with our patients and their families. We come to this understanding through reflection on the good or bad, acceptable or unacceptable experiences of our life and through exchanges with our colleagues and friends.

It is not always recognised that by giving due weight to the social, cultural and spiritual setting from which our patients are reaching their decisions and contrasting these to our own values – something we do on a daily basis – we are already employing an ethical framework to support the decision-making process. Gregory's description of the behaviour required of a physician demonstrates how one's own moral context is inevitably integrated into practice. Ethical teaching grounded in a clinical setting helps the healthcare professional define and understand his own moral context. A guide such as this text, which clearly and understandably works through the steps used to create a framework, is an essential part of supporting this understanding.

In a climate of rapidly growing medical advances in which the capacity to sustain life is ever greater, healthcare professionals are required to take responsibility for very complex clinical situations, particularly those involved in addressing end-of-life issues. There is often an added pressure on palliative care specialists who are called on as the experts to advise and support their clinical colleagues with these difficult decisions. Their help is recruited when others are considering when a move of treatment from curative to palliative intent is appropriate, and when a decision to withhold or withdraw treatment completely should be made. There is a continuing need for educational material which will provide a basis of information and example for the clinician facing these issues.

People will learn in a variety of ways, but one of the most immediate and relevant is by the use of example in circumstances that are recognisable and close to their own day-to-day experience. A formal lecture on the ethical aspects of an end-of-life decision-making process is undoubtedly a valid educational tool, but the opportunity to discuss and reflect on clinical examples gives the clinician the chance to review his own moral values. It helps him to recognise how much he may effect the information and the support communicated to the patient who is attempting to reach valid and acceptable decisions, and how he may temper this effect.

Ethical thought is integral to all aspects of medicine and especially to the implementation of palliative treatments that so crucially impact on a patient's quality of life. Health related ethical issues have recently assumed greater prominence in the political, legal and wider societal settings of our lives and there is a broader duty on clinicians to engage in the continuing debate on these fundamental concepts. This duty can only be managed from a basis of clearer understanding of these ethical principles.

Dr Teresa Tate
Medical Adviser to Marie Curie Cancer Care
Consultant in Palliative Medicine, Barts and the London NHS Trust
April 2005

About the authors

Roger Worthington lectures in medical law and ethics at the School of Medicine, Keele University, having previously been a lecturer at St George's Hospital Medical School (University of London). He is an advisor on standards and ethics at the General Medical Council (UK) and a Fellow of the Royal Society of Medicine.

Formerly in practice as an osteopath, he went on to gain an MA in medical ethics from Keele University and a PhD in philosophy from the State University of New York at Buffalo, USA. His research interests are in jurisprudence and the ethics of public policy, and ethical issues around the end of life. His first book is on Eastern philosophy, and the subject of his next book is medicine, ethics and multiculturalism.

Paddy Stone was educated at Wimbledon College, Gonville and Caius College, Cambridge and St Bartholomew's Hospital, London. He qualified in 1990 and obtained the MRCP in 1993 and his MD in cancer-related fatigue in 1999. Since July 2001 he has been the MacMillan Senior Lecturer in Palliative Medicine at St George's Hospital Medical School and Honorary Consultant at St George's Hospital NHS Trust. He has been a member of the Association of Palliative Medicine since 1993 and is currently the Secretary of the Palliative Care Research Society (UK). In 1997 he won the BMA Joan Dawkins Bursary to present his research at the BMA clinical conference in San Francisco. In 2000 he won the Association of Palliative Medicine Research award for his studies into cancer-related fatigue.

He runs the hospital support team at St George's Hospital, providing advice and support for inpatients with advanced and progressive disease. He also teaches on under-graduate and post-graduate courses at St George's Hospital Medical School. At the medical school he leads a small multidisciplinary research team. He is currently undertaking research into the mechanisms of cancer-related fatigue, methods to improve prognostic estimates for patients with advanced cancer, and the measurement of quality of life in a palliative care context.

Andrew Thorns is a consultant in palliative medicine holding a joint post between Pilgrims Hospice in Thanet and the Queen Elizabeth the Queen Mother Hospital. He also holds an honorary senior lecturer position at the University of Kent at Canterbury and participates in the running of the MSc in Supportive and Palliative Care which is based there. He has a keen interest in ethical issues at the end of life, in particular the use of sedation and opioids and the place of cardiopulmonary resuscitation. He is a member of the Ethics Committee of the Association for Palliative Medicine.

To all those who work with and care for people who are terminally ill, and who strive to meet their needs.

Part One

Chapter 1

Introduction to ethics at the end of life

Palliative care has now become established as a discrete area in clinical medicine, with dedicated clinical teams working in hospice settings, in the community and in hospitals, alongside clinical colleagues in oncology and other specialties. Palliative care ethics is of particular interest in that it brings into sharp focus important aspects of patient-centred care and critical decision making. The type of decisions made in this setting are different in nature from those dealing with more acute branches of medicine where, for instance, radical interventions are being considered. Some decisions intrinsically demand evaluative-type reasoning, where clinical aspects of care have to be carefully balanced against patients' expressed or perceived wishes or beliefs. By the time the palliative care team has been called in, opportunities for active intervention may have passed, but the palliative specialist nonetheless contributes to the debate about when that point has been reached.[1]

There are several different dynamics working in palliative decision-making scenarios. There is the dynamic of the relationship between the palliative physician and the multiprofessional team; there is also the dynamic of the relationship with the patient and the patient's family, both of which call on special skills, not all of which are strictly clinical. The implication is that members of the palliative care team can potentially have more to contribute if they are aware of the range of issues in play at a given point in time, and many of these have strong ethical components.

Rationales for clinical decision making include both medical and ethical criteria. The ethics of critical decision making can no more be separated from clinical circumstances surrounding a particular case than a medical decision can be viewed independently of its ethical implications. The point at which ethics is integrated into clinical practice may not always be reached, but it is still a worthwhile goal towards which to aspire.[2] Against this background there is nothing more poignant than managing the circumstances surrounding the final stages of a person's life, irrespective of the age of the patient or the profile of their disease.

The scope of palliative care ethics is surprisingly broad, and while this book provides critical analysis and commentary on some important topics, it cannot claim to be exhaustive in its scope. What it does do is address a subject that is not in any way static, and while some chapters should stand the test of time, such as Chapter 2 on ethical theory, others are a reflection on things as they seem at the time to the editor and to the contributors – the timeline being England and Wales in 2004 unless otherwise stated. Although such limitations are unavoidable, topics discussed could have wider applications, such as arguments about euthanasia and physician-assisted suicide (recognising that *legal* frameworks differ according to jurisdiction).

When it comes to definitions, the question of 'what is palliative care?' should be considered first, and an accepted definition is as follows:

The active total care of patients whose disease is not responsive to curative treatment. Control of pain, of other symptoms and of psychological, social and spiritual problems is paramount. The goal of palliative care is achievement of the best quality of life for patients and their families.

(WHO, 1990)

The 'palliative care approach' can be summarised as being an integral part of good clinical practice; affirming life, regarding dying as a normal process; neither hastening nor postponing death; providing relief from pain and other distressing symptoms, and integrating the psychological and spiritual aspects of care.[3]

At this stage it is also important to consider what is meant by the terms 'law' and 'ethics', which is not as obvious as might at first appear. The following may be said to underlie the ensuing text.

- The definition of the term 'law' depends on the field of application, e.g. law enforcement and practical jurisprudence, law making, and law as an expression of justice. In performing these roles, law is concerned with maintaining social order, dispensing corrective and retributive justice (in respect of civil and criminal branches of the law), the practical administration of the courts, the passing of new laws and the amendment and abolition of old ones, and with analysing the nature of justice itself and defining its social and political domains. No single definition can capture all these different aspects, but it is the philosophy of law and domains of justice that are of primary concern here.
- The term 'ethics' denotes an area of philosophy that has to do with moral codes and with individual or collective notions of right and wrong. Ethics and morals are synonymous, differing only in their modes of application.[4]

The book is organised into two parts. The first aims to provide an introduction to ethical and rights theory, and to address the question of making difficult decisions, especially those likely to be encountered in the palliative care setting, such as appropriate uses of sedation. The second part has just one aim, namely to provide examples for information and discussion on how these matters arise within the context of actual clinical cases. While no serious attempt is made to summarise material that appears later on, it is worth trying to provide a basic outline to guide the reader around the text, and to give an idea of what to expect and when. This opening chapter mainly attempts to provide some background and 'to set out the stall'.

Chapter Two offers an interpretation of ethical theory. The main subject matter of the book being applied medical ethics and not 'pure' philosophy, it makes little sense to try and provide anything resembling a history of ethics. Nonetheless, there is a historical component to this chapter, and although there are inevitably some gaps, the reader should gain something of a background perspective and begin to become familiar with concepts such as metaphysics, teleology and utility.

Ethics is sometimes viewed as a branch of philosophy, but it could also be argued that it is its core, because it concerns itself with the moral foundations of all human thought and behaviour. To make the material reasonably accessible it has been divided up by systems of thought, making it easier to refer back to when analysing the clinical cases in Part Two, and it would not be surprising if for many this chapter comprised a first attempt at reading ethics *or* philosophy. Full references are provided throughout, along with suggested further reading, explanations of unfamiliar words, and an eclectic list of prominent philosophers and ethicists.

The analysis of ethical theories does not just comprise a summary of other people's work; instead, the chapter draws on the editor's own research and is to an extent original (insofar as any philosophy is ever truly 'original'). As with many subjects, medical ethics at an introductory level is prone to generalisations, and this can sometimes result in compromises, but whether or not such pitfalls have been avoided here is something the reader will have to decide. Hopefully, the chapter will stimulate further thought and possibly further reading around the subject.

Chapter Three has its origins in a chapter on decision making written for *Ethical Issues in Palliative Care* (Webb, 2005), and while that chapter has some material in common, its central theme is different. In the Webb chapter the emphasis is on consent and the use of frameworks for critical decision making. Here, the emphasis is on models of decision making and their general applicability in the clinical environment. Material retained from the earlier version has been modified and expanded to provide a slightly fuller explanation of what these models are, and how they might or might not work in an applied setting. Some models are mathematically derived, such as game theory and the concept of equilibrium, but the analysis remains philosophical. For instance, the reasoning process in this last instance entails establishing whether there are benefits to be gained from seeking to establish equilibrium within the decision-making matrix. Formal logic is also mathematical in terms of the way it operates, but in the present context, it makes sense to focus more on logical analysis, as that is more meaningful in relation to how decision-making models can be applied. Logical argument, in terms of how it is both constructed and utilised, is certainly worthy of being retained and put to use.

Legal theory is then reintroduced (following on from preliminary explanations in Chapter Two) to try and explain *why* it has validity in ethical deliberations. Collective models of decision making, including democratic justice and the workings of multiprofessional teams, are also addressed and the latter seems to have particular relevance in relation to the ethics of palliative care.[5] In seeking to answer the question 'In what way can theoretical models of decision making be applied in a clinical setting?' the direction of movement is from a humanity-type focus to a science-based focus, taking in professional issues to do with roles and responsibilities along the way.

Chapter Four deals with the difficult issue of euthanasia, as well as topics falling under the general heading of withdrawing and withholding treatment, such as orders for or against resuscitation, and the doctrine of double effect. When discussing physician-assisted suicide there is no attempt to be directly provocative, but neither is there an attempt to smooth over the issues. They are dealt with frankly and in a way that is designed to be informative and useful for stimulating further discussion. Directly confronting issues dealing with death is never easy, even where it comprises part of professional working life. These topics have to be addressed without fear while being responsive to matters such as people's perceptions of 'death with dignity' and what is meant by 'a good death'. On balance the view is taken that euthanasia and physician-assisted suicide are not endorsed as appropriate ways to deal with important issues that relate to care of patients at the end of life.

The topic of rights is addressed in **Chapter Five**, together with analysis of the role, significance and potential limitations of patient autonomy, and how they fit into the patient–doctor relationship. Some broad questions about rights are first introduced in order to preface discussion about rights at the end of life, including topical issues to do with human rights legislation. Loose talk about rights often finds its way into media-type discussion about healthcare in general, and about the right to receive various forms of treatment. Careful scrutiny is needed to be able to establish the validity of rights-based claims, as well as possible implications for the patient and for the community as a whole. The National Institute for Clinical Excellence recently issued guidance on the provision of palliative care services, and in reviewing suggestions contained in this document, the opportunity is taken to try and clarify policy issues to do with decision making, rights and consent (NICE, 2004).

Here, as is often the case, ethics benefits from separate consideration away from the law. As part of this analysis, questions of conflicting autonomy, for example, between that which is patient centred and that which protects the rights of the professional, are worked through using case examples. In so doing it is hoped that a basic understanding can be reached as to the nature and purpose of rights in general and healthcare rights and autonomy in particular.

Sedation is an important research topic in palliative care with clinical, legal and ethical implications. It merits consideration as a topic in itself, and **Chapter Six** addresses it from each of these different perspectives. Discussion has to do with clinical control of levels of pain, as well as ethical implications of decreased patient awareness, and reduced powers to give or withhold consent following the clinical use of sedation. Specific areas of consent are worked through within the clinical setting, as well as practical issues such as what constitutes sedation, how and when sedation should be used, and what its primary purpose is meant to be. None of these questions are at all obvious, and the overall aim is for clarification resulting from analyses based on a detailed review of the literature. The doctrine of double effect and the role and usefulness of advance directives were first raised in Chapter Four but receive further consideration here on account of their practical relevance. While statutory legislation likely to come into effect soon will have practical implications,[6] this anticipated change in the law should not invalidate the arguments that are presented, either here or in other chapters.

Part Two of the book has one main aim: to illustrate material from previous chapters, and to allow readers and students to work through and discuss some fairly detailed cases. These cases have had a minimum of modification for the purpose of preserving the anonymity of former patients; in all other respects they have come directly off the wards. Included in the histories is a step-by-step commentary by a palliative care consultant. The editor has then added footnotes highlighting the ethical components of each case, and linking them with earlier material in the book (i.e. adding a sub-commentary from the point of view of a 'disinterested' third party taking the role of an ethics specialist or consultant). All the cases involve cancer patients, and although this is not uncommon in the palliative care setting, it is nonetheless recognised that patients coming under the care of such teams may have other conditions. In other respects the cases vary considerably, and the narratives can simply be allowed to speak for themselves.

Notes to Chapter 1

1   This point is well illustrated in Case 3 in Part Two.
2   Cf. Hattab (2004) for an evaluation of the role of ethics teaching in medical education in an international setting.
3   The principles of palliative care are accepted as incorporating the following:
    * focus on quality of life which includes good symptom control
    * whole person approach
    * care which encompasses both the individual and those that matter to them
    * respect for patient autonomy
    * emphasis on open and sensitive communication.
    Cf. WHO (1990). For further information on palliative care principles and philosophy see: Doyle *et al.* (1998).
4   Philosophically, the relationship between law and ethics is both dynamic and fluid, each exerting an influence over the other. An element of symbiosis would be seen as reflecting a healthy relationship between these two concepts that only sometimes intersect to a point where they occupy the same domains.
5   Topics do not appear in this order within the chapter itself.
6   Cf. the Mental Capacity Bill 2004.

Chapter 2

An explanation of ethical theory

Ethics and morals

The words 'ethics' and 'morals' have a common meaning, ethics merely coming from the Greek and morals coming from the Latin. Although they share a definition and modern usage favours the Greek over the Latin in the general context of professionalism, it is worth remembering that as soon as one begins to do ethical analysis the subject under discussion is morals. When it comes to applied ethics, context does have a bearing in that not all philosophical argument takes place in the abstract. Applied ethics covers a range of topics, and almost by definition it can be employed by non-experts, albeit with some degree of training. Rather than claim ownership of a body of knowledge, the professional philosopher (or ethicist) may well act in the role of facilitator or expert advisor.

As a subject, law and ethics is now part of the normal curriculum in medical education, and this fairly recent development is certainly welcome. Clinicians need to be equipped to deal with moral conflicts that arise in the context of modern clinical practice. Such conflicts may well challenge one's ethical understanding, and in the case of the palliative care professional, ethics plays an important role in the context of decision making, planning and care giving. The philosopher and clinician may share in the processes of deliberation, but clinicians work either alone or as part of a team with other healthcare professionals, i.e. not normally with a philosopher. Thus at a practical level the healthcare professional needs to be able to make use of a grounding in ethics, performing independent judgements and looking for help when and where it is needed. This chapter will try and fill some gaps in terms of providing this ethical grounding.

It should be remembered that applied ethics affects people's lives, not just potentially at some point in the future, but 'here and now' in hospitals, in hospices and in the community. Ethics is not just a search for a fix when something goes wrong, neither is it necessarily about constructing elaborate hypotheses. It is about helping influence decisions as they are made with the aim of promoting social welfare in general, and the welfare of particular others (i.e. patients), as well as helping minimise or mitigate the effects of medically induced harm. Resolving a clinical ethical dilemma involves weighing things in the balance to assess one set of risks against another, a known benefit against an unknown risk, a known risk against an uncertain benefit, and/or being able to balance competing moral values. In order to be able to perform or even attempt to perform these tasks, the healthcare professional needs something to which s/he can refer.

Ethical analysis is an evaluative process, not an exact science, and so there are no ready-made answers; each case needs to be assessed on its merits in relation to the available information. If it were simply a question of benchmarking and comparing the presenting facts against a clearly defined set of values, there would be no need for philosophy at all. Difficult decisions could be left to someone in a position of authority or simply handed over to legal experts. The relationship between law and morality is not without interest; for now, suffice it to say that for something to be moral, it will not necessarily be in accord with the law. Similarly, for something to be legal, it will not automatically be in accord with moral codes of society. Multicultural society does not have an absolute or universal moral code; it has sets of beliefs that have their origin in a range of cultural values that may or may not be reflected in the law. Some argue it is necessary that in order for something to be enshrined in law, it must be based on moral belief or that for something to be moral it is sufficient that it be in accord with the law. But matters are not that simple, and since the advent of the positivist tradition various challenges have been made towards these assumptions.

First, it is time for a brief look back into history to see where ideas such as positivism, utilitarianism and Kantianism came from and what they mean to the modern healthcare professional. Ethics assumes a major role in the history of Western philosophy, and it is broadly concerned with how one should live, as well as (but not limited to) how one should practise medicine. In classical times the subject of ethics ranged from Pythagorean metaphysics to Socratic dialogues and to the natural theories of Galen, to say nothing of the historical importance of the Hippocratic tradition or of Aristotelian ethics. But to attempt to trace the evolution of ethical thought would take an entire volume and it is more appropriate here to trace the history of ethical concepts than the history of ethics itself.

Introducing metaphysics

While this may be a challenging method of doing philosophical analysis, metaphysics is a good place to start in that it can help furnish useful tools for analysing difficult situations that do not resolve themselves by using other methods. The term 'metaphysics' is ontological, i.e. one that concerns itself with the nature of how things are rather than what things do. The prefix 'meta' is a reminder that the scope of the term is necessarily broad; the word 'physics' can be misleading in that physics normally describes one of the so-called hard sciences. Metaphysics, on the other hand, is about concepts and abstractions and so it is not something on which a strict empiricist may want to spend long in that it explores a somewhat different way of thinking.

Metaphysical analysis may not be capable of arriving at concrete proof for any given proposition or assertion; instead what it aims to do is consider a proposition from angles that differ from those relating to merely epistemic (knowledge-based) concerns. In short, metaphysics is about how things really are and not merely how they seem to be. Knowledge that is restricted to material facts is incomplete insofar as it does not take account of things that are hidden from view. Metaphysics, therefore, is about the 'inner workings' of material substance, by which I do not mean sub-atomic, molecular, genetic or other scientific ways of analysing matter. Metaphysical knowledge is about the 'essence' of a thing, not the thing itself, and examining a proposition in terms of metaphysics can mean stretching the mind in ways to which it might not be accustomed. While this may be discomforting, it can be revealing when it comes to making evaluative-type judgments.

To take a clinical example, issues surrounding quality of life are often metaphysical in nature, i.e. having more to do with qualitative than with quantitative-type analysis. The concept of quality-adjusted life years (QALYs) offers a formulaic approach towards evaluations at the end of life, and while it may seem strange to talk about QALYs in a context of introducing metaphysics, a good way to gain a handle on something is by describing its opposite. Plenty of examples of this method of explanation can be found in philosophical discourse.

Take a medical intervention such as combination chemotherapy that is expensive to administer and may only lead to a short extension of life. The associated risks of treatment are quite high, the quality of life during treatment is usually poor, and the number of years of life gained may just be measured in fractions. However, *not* to treat a cancer patient with chemotherapy may be quite wrong, even though it would reduce the cost of treatment and the risk of treatment itself. Life extension is nil if the patient dies from the underlying condition, either before or during treatment. But quality of life in the remaining weeks or months matters a great deal, and though the final outcome may still be death, the trade-off between risks and benefits may be better measured in qualitative than in quantitative terms. A metaphysical-type judgment would focus more on quality of life, and about which set of values is applicable in an end-of-life situation. Metaphysical considerations can be highly relevant, and arguments couched in terms of QALYs tend to deny the subtle characteristics of a situation. Not surprisingly, QALYs are often used in making decisions about resource allocation, which clearly lend themselves to quantitative methods of analysis. There is nothing metaphysical about QALYs, and so patient-centred value judgments are much more likely to benefit from the inclusion of metaphysical analysis as part of the reasoning process.

Ethics in ancient Greece

Going back in time, a school of philosophy that can be traced back to ancient Greece is that founded by Pythagoras. It was well suited to metaphysical analysis, even though Pythagoras himself achieved greater fame in respect of his science of mathematics. Interestingly, his metaphysics drew inspiration from the East, and the Pythagorean School was unique in its time, forming a bridge between the classical teaching of ancient civilisations of India and Greece. Unfortunately, though, little recorded information from that time survives, largely because of having attracted the attention of the 'sceptics', a hard-headed group that viewed metaphysics with suspicion and set about burning anything that resembled Pythagorean thought. Fortunately, modern philosophers attack each other by different means, but the Pythagorean School is still rather shrouded in mystery. Aristotelian metaphysics has survived, even though the 14 books that comprise the volume *Metaphysics* are difficult to read, even in translation, and it is open to many differences in interpretation.[1] Nonetheless, *Metaphysics* forms an important ontological treatise and it has generated a large quantity of secondary literature. Better known and far more widely read is

Aristotle's *Nicomachean Ethics*, sometimes known simply as 'The Ethics', and in it Aristotle discusses at length ideas such as virtue, justice, happiness and rationality. Study of this work has given rise to something known as the 'eudaimonic method', in which happiness and rationality are related to moral virtue and excellence (an interesting precursor to later utilitarian systems of thought).

A well-known classical method of teaching philosophy is to use the Socratic method. Technically this is known as the 'elenchic method'[2] and it comprises a dialogue in which the questioner is asked to express a point of view that is then countered by the master, in this case Socrates, as recorded in the writings of Plato in the early *Dialogues*. The method is akin to asking a student to express an ethical opinion and then pointing out the errors in their reasoning. It is especially powerful if the person offering an opinion is a so-called expert and the philosopher is able to refute that argument (as Socrates was known to have enjoyed doing). While the method has the appearance of a sophisticated form of sport, it is recognised as a way of highlighting contentious issues such as those presenting in the form of moral dilemmas.

In the *Apology*, Plato argues famously that 'an unexamined life is not worth living'.[3] It is here that Socrates upholds the importance of virtue as an ideal worth living for, and in this late work the tone is generally more constructive than in the earlier elenchic dialogues. This time the listener is exhorted to listen to an explanation in support of a method of reasoning about the importance of moral virtue and the soul, and this method can be used in a modern context with peer pressure exerting the kind of influence once considered the prerogative of the master. Didactic teaching assumes a lesser importance in relation to modern methods of teaching and learning, but a meaningful dialogue, prompted by carefully chosen remarks, offers a constructive method of engaging students in interactive discussion. The Socratic method thus can be adapted to suit different needs and situations.

Teleology (Aristotle, Aquinas and beyond)

If something has a particular attribute such as colour, shape or form, the inherent characteristics are what they are 'by nature', hence teleological. If the characteristics of a thing are the result of man-made fashioning then they are no longer by nature but 'assumed'. In scientific terms, to describe the genetic composition of an organism (including a human organism) is one way of describing its inner nature. On the other hand, to describe the characteristics that come under the heading 'phenotype' would be to consider how an organism interacts with the environment or how someone behaves as an individual.[4] Other things, such as the physical nature of the universe and genotypical characteristics, are simply 'the way they are', i.e. independently of how they are perceived. This does not rule out the possibility of subtle interactions (such as between genotype and phenotype) but in terms of identity, a given object or organism is best described teleologically by reference to its inner nature.

In the *Nicomachean Ethics* Aristotle talks about the nature of bronze and its inherent characteristics once formed into a shape, such as the sculpture of an individual or thing. Bronze is an alloy so it does not occur 'in nature', but there is a difference between a lump of bronze and a work of art in which the bronze is fashioned in a particular way. Some philosophy applies this type of reasoning to law and morals, in which 'by nature' is substituted and taken to mean 'ordained by God'. Such reasoning was certainly used by Aquinas, for whom there was never much sense of moral ambiguity; if something was wrong by nature, it contradicted God's laws and was not therefore subject to ordinary rationalisation.[5]

Aristotle and Aquinas both made teleological observations about substance and universal matter, but one could infer from their theologies that their observations would have had very different meanings. Aristotle was a rationalist and greatly admired the powers of the human intellect but nonetheless continued to argue that many things were the way they were simply 'by nature'. For example, a farmer tends his fields because it is his natural disposition to so do; physicians care for their patients in the same way, as it would be against their inner nature not to do so. For Aristotle, who was no atheist, such inner nature was something with which (or into which) one was born; for Aquinas it was more a question of divine grace and provenance.

For centuries, the institution of the church came to hold power over scientific and philosophical discourse, and, for example, being admitted to the church was once a precondition of taking up an appointment at Cambridge. Newton, as it happens, steadfastly refused to do this, even though he eventually took up rooms. He went on to use those rooms in Cambridge to perform alchemical experiments, which predated his more famous scientific discoveries.[6] When it came to church law, alchemy was considered much more heretical than 'science', which enjoyed a measure of respectability that never was afforded to alchemy. Some things clearly were best not discussed too openly.

Rationality and teleology need not be in opposition to one another, even when premised on quite different assumptions. An empiricist would not want to suspend belief in the material world, as based on empirical observation (i.e. 'facts' capable of scientific proof). Galileo Galilei employed both rationality and empirical observation to describe how things were in space and the universe (notably, without recourse to religious authorities of the time). Only recently did the Roman Catholic Church apologise for having persecuted Galileo, and while neither politics nor religion is being discussed here, there is real historical tension between established systems of belief and the threat posed by empirically driven observation. Such forces were so powerful that in no way could they be ignored. Nonetheless, to say that something is how it is 'by nature' is not philosophically interesting because it does not say very much other than that a thing is what it is, either as a matter of personal belief and/or that it can be verified by empirical observation. It therefore has limited value in relation to moral discourse.

Descartes, a 'classical' empiricist from the early modern era, was criticised by many philosophers (Newton in particular) for being a dualist, and for suggesting that mind and body were of a different nature. But the identities of mind, brain and consciousness are still often confused and while Western philosophy tends to connect mind with brain, it has little to offer by way of explanation for what is meant by the term 'consciousness' (simply described by Descartes as an 'activity of the soul'). The brain is a physical entity capable of a degree of proof as to its anatomical identity, and its attributes as an organ can be accurately described in neurological terms. But philosophically, mind cannot be described in the same way,[7] and Descartes could not accept that all aspects of mind and consciousness were capable of being equated with the physical human brain. Even though the attentions of Leibnitz, Newton and Gassendi and others resulted in rejection of most of Descartes' hypotheses, Cartesian philosophy nonetheless had a profound influence on this important period of history known as the Enlightenment.

Kantian ethics

Kant's notion of respect for persons and respect for bodily integrity is antecedent to modern notions of rights and patient autonomy.[8] Kantian ethics, which unlike utilitarianism is *non-consequentialist*, upholds the moral signifi-cance of the nature of an act as of greater importance than the final outcome. Kant offers a quintessentially *deontological* perspective, with an implicit belief in the existence of moral imperatives underlying his critical thinking.[9] To use his own words:

> We know our own freedom (from which all moral laws and hence all rights as well as duties are derived) only through the moral impera-tive, which is a proposition commanding duties. The capacity to obligate others to a duty, that is, the concept of a right, can be subse-quently derived from this imperative.
>
> (Ladd, 1999: Part 1)

Kant's thinking has been highly influential in the evolution of Western thought. It served as a touchstone for early bioethical analysis and still holds sway for many ethicists, particularly in the United States. Kant's ideals were based on an assumption of personal religious belief; at the same time they were highly sophisticated and tempered by strong rational intellectualism. While like any theory, Kantian theory has its limitations, it cannot be dismissed, and his person-centred approach to ethical reasoning lies at the core of many modern theories of rights and obligations.

When it comes to discussions about healthcare, Kantian theory is unable to justify a right to healthcare beyond a duty to rescue, and Kant's preoccupation with the rights of the individual can sometimes be at the expense of the wider interests of a community. But the greatest inherent difficulty with Kantian ethics is its dependence upon what are known as *a priori* categorical imperatives (previously existing moral absolutes), which presuppose the existence of commonly held views in terms of social attitude and values. While certain assumptions can reasonably have been made with regard to late eighteenth-century German social conditions, the same cannot be said in respect of today's multicultural, pluralist society. Furthermore, separating means from ends is potentially as harmful as attaching over-riding significance to ends irrespective of how they are achieved. It is difficult to justify the quality of an act if it results in otherwise avoidable harm. Similarly, a fixation on final outcome can blind one to the suffering of known or unknown 'others' along the way. Neither method is desirable on its own, and any method of analysis capable of holding one in balance with the other (i.e. means versus ends) would have a strong moral appeal. There is a large body of primary or secondary literature relating to Kantian ethics, but what is of particular interest in the present context is the flourishing neo-Kantian school, on which much bioethical discussion has come to be based.

Twentieth-century deontology

John Rawls, who died in 2002, was a strong defender and leading exponent of modern liberal democratic theory based on neo-Kantian ideals. He was a contractarian, and his ethical principles were based on the premiss of social choice made from behind a so-called 'veil of ignorance', that is, a type of 'original position' untempered by social custom, class or privilege. The device theoretically ensured that social decisions were made in the abstract from a hypothetical position of isolation, thereby ensuring that 'no one is advantaged or disadvantaged in the choice of principles by the outcome of natural chance or the contingency of social circumstances' (Rawls, 2001: Chapter 1.3). His theories earned him fame within the academic community, as well as a great deal of well-informed criticism (which for a philosopher can be construed as a 'plus' by having one's ideas taken seriously and widely disseminated).

Kantian ethics is based on assumptions relating to the existence of moral absolutes; Rawlsian ethics is even more specific, based on a deductive system whereby all ethical principles are derived from two moral principles that need to be treated as fixed points. They are these, namely that:

> (1) Each person is to have an equal right to the most extensive total system of equal basic liberties compatible with a similar system of liberty for all;
> (2) Social and economic inequalities are to be arranged so that they are both a) to the greatest benefit of the least advantaged, consistent with the just savings principles, and b) attached to offices and positions open to all under conditions of fair equality of opportunity.
> (Rawls, 2001: Chapter 5.46)

The second principle is to be fully dependent upon acceptance of the first, although it should be remembered that the argument for equal rights is not about material wealth or economic parity but so-called 'equality of opportunity'. This is a reasonable ideal if impossible to actuate because conditions of equality are not inherent in ordinary society, and because it is impossible to ignore the social reality of people's individual circumstances and their rights to make autonomous choices. Equality of opportunity may not be an ethically appropriate ideal because it raises too many questions about the fairness of how that end ought to be achieved, and it inevitably restrains personal choice.

Rawlsian ethics demands redistribution of resources in the direction of the least well-off, without qualification as to how much wealth is to be transferred and upon what premiss, other than to satisfy an ideal. Social justice demands that an element of redistribution may be necessary in order to ensure, for example, that no sector of the population is without a basic level of healthcare provision. But redistribution only happens of its own volition in conditions of collective altruism or widespread agreement about who would benefit, to what extent and how (hence, not at all). Some element of coercion is considered essential, as in the case with systems of taxation whereby penalties exist for non-compliance and failure to pay what one owes to the government. But such coercion challenges Rawls' own theory of liberty, which claims that 'Everyone is assured an equal liberty to pursue whatever plan of life he pleases as long as it does not violate what justice demands' (Rawls, 2001: Chapter 2.15). According to Rawls, anything that reduces liberty has to be justified in accordance with this premiss, which could make it difficult for governments to enact programmes of social welfare and reform, such as a widespread entitlement to healthcare service provision (unless there was first a broad agreement about the need for strong institutions in support of social justice).

Rawls admits to being indebted to Kant for the inspiration of his ethical ideals. He propounds a deontological system of rights and obligations that continue to attract interest and controversy in equal measure. His magnum opus, *The Theory of Justice* (1971), unfortunately does not comprise a recipe for applied ethics by reason of being dependent on purely abstract hypotheses. Rawls says almost nothing about health or healthcare, and contents himself with categorising them under a general heading of 'natural goods', forming part of a list of social goods and values afforded the general status of a 'right'. Under the scheme he classes health, vigour, intelligence and imagination together under one heading, thereby giving them less weight than the primary goods of rights, liberty and opportunities. This scheme, combined with the 'difference principle' (meant to describe the conditions under which it is considered just to redistribute assets within society), forms the main ethic behind his notion of distributive justice. However, as Sen argues, 'the primary goods approach seems to take little note of the diversity of human beings',[10] and this notion of diversity is too important to ignore.

Ronald Dworkin, a contemporary of Rawls, is best known for his critique of HLA Hart's philosophy of law (Hart, 1964), and in *Law's Empire* (1986) he argues against Hart's brand of legal positivism. In a more recent work, *Sovereign Virtue* (2000), Dworkin concerns himself with the ethics of virtue, and this book contains many bioethical topics of discussion. In it Dworkin gives an account of social justice and how things might be if society in general was less marked by social inequalities. This endeavour seems reasonable enough, but equity and fairness provide better tools for making critical judgments about moral and social values than hypothesis based on an artificially construed form of social equality.

Equity and equality are not the same, and while both are difficult to define in absolute terms, it can lead to philosophical confusion to avoid making a distinction. For example, equal shares of goods and services may or may not be fair depending on how equality is achieved, and how successful it is in balancing the rights of individuals (e.g. for someone to enjoy the fruits of their own labour) against broader community-based rights. Equity is better suited to ethical analysis than equality, because apart from anything else, equality is politically laden in that it does not happen without state intervention and a significant redistribution of social goods and services.

Richard Posner, a contemporary of Dworkin, an academic and a well-known appellate judge in the USA, has little time for the theories of Rawls, Dworkin or

Hart, and he provides a strong critique of academic jurisprudence as well as American legal education and its associated scholarly institutions (Posner, 2002). Posner attempts to demystify legal theory, and at the same time to critique contemporary legal scholarship, including all prevalent forms of legal positivism. If nothing else, Posner offers a very different perspective on legal theory, by insisting that moral theory is incapable of bringing anything useful to the debate about the role of law in society and how lawyers conduct their judicial business. He advocates that law should be 'steered by the light of pragmatism', which, even though his general criticisms are harsh, is a point well made in that an element of pragmatism is a useful tool for avoiding extremes as regards the role and function of law.

The extent to which pragmatism has a place in ethical debate is itself not without contention. For the idealist, and for anyone asserting the importance of moral imperatives, pragmatism has no place in that for such a person actions must be seen in terms of right and wrong, not what is (or is not) expedient at a given point in time. In that many clinical ethical dilemmas involve making decisions based on the specifics of a given case, it would be impossible to rule out all pragmatic considerations. Some constraints simply cannot be avoided, and limiting factors impinge on the realities of much clinical decision making.[11] Pragmatism, however, can also be spelt with a capital 'P', and in this case it is taken to refer to a school of American thought in the early twentieth century. Names such as James, Royce and Dewey are associated with a movement that was very influential in establishing bioethics as a serious subject of study.

Pragmatism is seen by some as too permissive, allowing principles to be sacrificed and moral idealism ignored. But that need not be the case, and in the passage quoted here a sense of vision becomes evident in the attempt to incorporate ethical ideals into making practical decisions:

> What is ethical practice? It is embracing ambiguity and uncertainty while eschewing paternalistic expertise and attitudes and courageously seeking to deliver quality and reasonable healthcare to those who need it. It is applying the principle of proportionality in a context of interpretation and community building that requires honesty, humility, and loyalty while seeking justice with courage and evincing an attitude of positive hope and expectation.[12]

It can certainly be argued that moral relativism does not fit within the context of legal decision making where a ruling has to be made one way or another in terms of the culpability (criminal or otherwise) of an individual or institution. However, legal scholarship can potentially inform the debate about moral philosophy and, as argued later on, can reliably inform the debate about what constitutes ethical conduct.

The concept of utility

It is time now to consider the principle of utility in order to provide the other half of the (consequentialist, non-consequentialist) equation. Kant's continental philosophy is in sharp contrast with JS Mill's English utilitarian theory, the latter being concerned primarily with achieving the greatest good for the greatest numbers of people, thus stressing ends rather than means. Mill was a student of Jeremy Bentham, and Bentham's theory of utility was based in part on the work of the Italian philosopher, Beccaria. Nothing is without precedent, although as far as utility is concerned we could effectively start in England in 1789 with the publication of *An Introduction to the Principles of Morals and Legislation* by Jeremy Bentham (Bentham, 1968). His definition of utility reads as follows:

> By the principle of utility is meant that principle which approves or disapproves of every action whatsoever, according to the tendency which it appears to have to augment or diminish the happiness of the party whose interest is in question: or, what is the same thing in other words, to promote or to oppose that happiness. I say of every action whatsoever; and therefore not only of every action of a private individual, but of every measure of government. [Chap 1.2]

Bentham is known for his contribution to jurisprudence and to political philosophy, and although Bentham's moral principles are intertwined with his theories of government and the law, his jurisprudence actually owes little to moral theory. Hart says that 'Bentham calls the principle of utility "the measure of right and wrong" and regards it as constituting the standards by which both the law and the conventional morality of any society should be judged' (Hart, 2001: p.86). However, Bentham's claim is overstated and cannot really be upheld.

The ethics of Bentham is essentially about public duty and obligation, but it is logically impossible on the one hand to pursue happiness and avoid pain, while on the other hand upholding the interests of the community as part of one's duty to the public. Such goals are in natural opposition, and Bentham has no viable formula for resolving the tensions that arise from this philosophical bind. Personal morality is a matter of individual conscience, premissed on one's sense of religious and/or social convictions. The pursuit of pleasure has nothing to do with public morality, and in fact may not have much to do with morality at all. Also, it is worth noting that Bentham's claim is quite different from that made by Aristotle, who argued that happiness came from the pursuit of excellence, and not that pleasure was a goal to seek for its own sake.

Utility, as designed to promote social welfare by increasing the sum of total happiness, is nonetheless portrayed as an altruistic philosophy promoting the needs of society over those of the individual. This may be the utilitarian ideal but for Bentham, social good was a by-product of maximising individual happiness, and his philosophy is hedonistic in that pleasure is to be sought as an end in itself, and pain is to be eschewed at all costs. It is not surprising that Bentham had a difficult task defending his ideals, especially against criticism from his arch-rival, Kant, who found such views so reactionary as to be 'likely to pervert public morals'.

Utility was to flourish at the hands of JS Mill, and his essay simply called *Utilitarianism* (first published in 1861) is a defining classic as regards this school of philosophy (Crisp, 1998). His primary definition of utility reads as follows:

> According to the greatest happiness principle ... the ultimate end,

with reference to and for the sake of which all other things are desirable – whether we are considering our own good or that of other people – is an existence exempt as far as possible from pain, and as rich as possible in enjoyments, both in point of quantity and quality. [Chap. 2]

Mill's account is still hedonistic but it shows greater recognition of the fact of human suffering and of the need to curtail individual liberty than that displayed by Bentham, even though in both cases the ultimate goal accords with the greatest happiness principle.

Mill was an empiricist, and for him it was better to form moral judgments based on assessment of the consequences of an act or intervention than to debate the merits and demerits of the nature of the act itself. Such debate would involve too much metaphysical and speculative analysis. However, Mill too lands himself in difficulties by making the assertion that utility is 'the ultimate appeal on all ethical questions'.[13] This is unproven and unsustainable, and is a distortion of reality in that it fails to recognise the possibility of competing ethical principles. For Mill, utility simply is *the* ethical principle.

Utilitarianism is sometimes split into act- and rule-utilitarianism, but this distinction serves only to highlight the contradictions inherent in Mill's philosophy, and not to clarify his ideals (Beauchamp, 1994: Chapter X). Put simply, a philosophical chain of reasoning cannot be inductive and deductive at the same time, act-utilitarianism being primarily inductive and concerned with the specifics of a particular case, and rule-utilitarianism being deductive, concerned with the broad application of moral principles. It is likely to generate confusion to try and sustain a distinction ('act' versus 'rule') that is so far from being watertight.

In the domain of criminal law and jurisprudence, utility falls into a trap of justifying punishment of the innocent if by so doing it promotes greater public adherence to the rule of law. It can also be partially blind to minority interests, because the greater good is not necessarily served by actively promoting the interests of minorities (although such interpretation ignores the fact that the whole can be served by attending to the needs of the constituent parts). Mill argued in defence of impartiality, but minority or disadvantaged groups often need compensatory mechanisms to help them compete in society or else they tend to lose out, and so impartiality may not be sufficient on its own. This is a classic case of a dichotomy often seen between defending the rights of the individual and defending the rights of the wider community, which is still playing out on the modern political stage.[14]

Mill's theory of correlative rights is incomplete, and his defence of individual liberty does not succeed in resolving tensions that so often arise between competing social interests. His essay *On Liberty* deals with this point at some length, and he describes how the state should intervene in a given situation, opting generally for minimal state interference. But by so doing Mill makes considerable demands on the individual and his/her general sense of morality, which may be over-optimistic as well as unrealistic.

Utility has another problem in that acting according to one set of ideals (i.e. utilitarian) almost inevitably brings one into conflict with different social ideals (e.g. deontological), and there are no ready formulae for dealing with such conflicts. Either the end result is what matters most or how an act is justified, and philosophically, it is very difficult to hold ends and means in a state of equilibrium.

Bernard Williams, a well-known critic of utilitarianism, writes:

> The demands of political reality and the complexities of political thought are obstinately what they are, and in face of them the simple-mindedness of utilitarianism disqualifies it totally.[15]

This view is unequivocal, and Mill's assertion that 'if utility is the ultimate source of moral obligations, utility may be invoked to decide between when their demands are incompatible' (Mills, 1984: Chapter 2) remains unproven. Utility is not a universal theory any more than deontology. Neither theory is capable of resolving all ethical dilemmas although each has its own merits.

Four principles

Something approaching a tradition has built up over the last 30 years which gives an elevated status to the four 'classic' principles of bioethics: *autonomy, justice, beneficence* and *non-maleficence*. The four principles method seeks to identify the ethical components of a case by relating them to one or more of the principles. It works on the premiss that there are such things as absolute moral principles, capable of indicating the most appropriate (or least inappropriate) course of action in a given situation.[16]

This is a deontological mode of reasoning, and what was a matter of necessity to Kant in terms of the importance attached to moral principles is different in the context of modern pluralist society, where space must be left to allow for different sets of values to coexist. In reality, each principle can find itself in opposition to one or more of the others, ultimately leaving the hard-working clinician with no useful guidance in terms of having to make a morally based decision.

Recognising that the four principles are widely talked about, the question of definitions needs to be addressed.

- **Autonomy** – this tends to be regarded as paramount and can be defined as:
  A state of being self-governing, e.g. when someone is able to exercise free will and liberty in making a personal (medical) decision. Autonomy allows patients the right to give or withhold consent to a particular intervention, be it a type of treatment (including surgery) or taking part in research. It is applicable to anyone who is legally competent.
- **Justice** – from Aristotle onwards, no philosopher has been able to sustain a single working definition of justice. However, for practical purposes it can be taken to mean the following (recognising that there are several different types of justice, such as civil, criminal, political, retributive, distributive, and corrective):
  An expression denoting conditions of fairness and equity. Something that can serve as a means of determining the allocation of resources amongst members of society, and provide a method of righting wrongs. That which

is upheld to protect citizens from the actions of others who engage in criminal or unjust behaviour.

- **Beneficence** – literally 'being charitable' or doing good, e.g.:
  Exercising duty of care so as to maximise patient well-being by exercising clinical judgment and going beyond standards set by legal minima. A beneficent physician may be said to be one who aspires towards virtue.
- **Non-maleficence** – doing no harm; i.e.:
  The avoidance of that which is likely to put persons at risk of an otherwise avoidable harm. A first step towards practical demonstration of beneficence, hence an ideal to which all physicians might aspire, as defined under the Hippocratic Oath.

Analytic jurisprudence

Jurisprudential and logical analysis may be capable of providing a viable, workable basis for making ethical decisions. In the case of medical ethics, jurisprudential reasoning refers to a method of analysis that focuses on the nature and function of the law (the investigation of legal process constituting a different type of jurisprudence). Unlike the 'principles', analytic jurisprudence is potentially capable of being flexible and socially inclusive. It is intellectually robust and, properly applied, can provide a firm foundation upon which to base ethical reasoning.

Law and morality are mutually supportive concepts, and neither necessity nor sufficiency is satisfied by failing to recognise differences between them. As has already been noted, context matters in applied ethics and in the translation from theory to practice, arguments do not take place in a void. It has rightly been said that 'the factual criteria for determining whether or not a proposition of law is true or false are indexed to particular legal systems, whereas the criteria for the semantic content of the concept of law are not' (Coleman, 2001). In short, what is or is not lawful depends on what is embodied in a particular legal system; morality, however, may not be so dependent.

For instance, it would be accurate to say that euthanasia is legal in the Netherlands, but it does not mean to say that every Dutch citizen thinks that euthanasia is moral. Neither does it mean that people living in Italy subscribe to a different code of morality simply because euthanasia is *illegal* in that country. Codes of morality operate at a number of different levels, ranging from personal to societal, all the way up to national and international levels, but boundaries of morality do not necessarily coincide with the boundaries of legality. Boundaries of legality are usually defined in relation to political justice, which needs to be part of a separate discussion.

Adherence to codes of morality and adherence to the law are not the same activity, albeit depending on interpretation of concepts such as validity, authority, legitimacy and enforceability. Thus, since codes of morality may or may not be in accord with the actual content of the law, there is a need for caution in adopting rules of dependence that link morality with legality. The expressions are neither interchangeable nor completely unrelated, and determining the basis of legality means considering a range of moral values, which in particular must recognise the fact of what may be termed 'natural social diversity'.

Upholding the rule of law is conducive to social stability, and individual members of society cannot generally be left to choose which laws to accept and which to ignore. While moral values are things which can be respected collectively or on an individual basis, the framework of the law is somewhat different in that while it may be binding on individuals, it is best defined in relation to society as a whole. In effect, law is a social reality interpreted and implemented by those with specialised knowledge (i.e. not by the general public).[17] If this is indeed the case, it is unethical to define the basis of law according to the interests of only one sector of the community, whether or not it is in a majority. To have moral validity, the law needs to be broad and socially inclusive.

Rights and personal identity

Two important topics have yet to be discussed:

1 what is a right and how should it be defined and
2 how to deal with questions of personal identity and establishing who, exactly, is meant to exercise autonomy, enjoy a right or bear a burden towards the satisfaction or fulfilment of a right in others.[18]

These concepts are of course closely intertwined. Some rights concern the individual, such as personal autonomy, and some concern a body of people, such as a profession, nation or group of nations (e.g. the European Union). Universal human rights are the business of international bodies such as the United Nations; other rights, such as those referred to in the Human Rights Act 1998, affect a whole population, but have nonetheless to be interpreted by the courts in order to define how rights are to be assigned or enjoyed by individual members of society.[19]

Individual autonomy defines the basis upon which a person decides whether or not s/he wants something to happen (or not to happen). Individual rights have some limits, as it does not make sense if the exercise of one person's autonomous rights directly impinges on the rights of another. In common with the four principles discussed earlier, rights can and do conflict with one another. One person's rights can conflict with another person's rights (e.g. between a patient exercising individual autonomy and his/her physician exercising professional autonomy, with each holding opposing views). Furthermore, individual rights can conflict with community rights and thus be detrimental to the rights and freedoms of others. Such matters are indeed complex and they call into question what it means to be 'a person'.

Philosophers have long debated what it means to be a person and, ethically speaking, much rides on the attribution of personhood. The debate surrounding the so-called 'right to die' highlights the importance of this point, and unless or until personhood can be satisfactorily defined, such disputes are set to continue. Society does not quite know whom it wants to treat as individuals (as persons) and when, and a patient in a deep or irreversible coma, for example, displays none of the characteristics normally associated with being a person. No single definition of personhood captures it entirely. However, an explanation offered by John Locke is useful and often quoted:

> [A Person is] a thinking intelligent Being, that has reason and reflection, and can consider it self as it self, the same thinking thing in different times and places, which it does only by that consciousness, which is inseparable from thinking, and it seems to be to it: It being impossible for any one to perceive, without perceiving, that he does perceive ... in this alone consists personal Identity, i.e., the sameness of a rational Being ... it being impossible to make personal Identity to consist in anything but consciousness. [sic]
>
> (Locke, 1979: Book 2: 27)

While Locke's use of language may seem strange, and this is but one paragraph from a very long work, this passage nonetheless has some relevance to the present enquiry.

Consciousness is 'that which perceives', i.e. the very essence of a person, so in order to better understand what it means to be a person, the question of consciousness has first to be addressed. Locke says nothing about the organ 'brain', the senses of perception or rational thought at this point; he talks instead about perception and identity predicating a form of critical self-awareness. But this interpretation is open to a charge of dualism in that it begs the question 'can a person perceive him/herself without being two beings, or without there being some kind of higher and lower consciousness?'. But having degrees of consciousness is not an impossible abstraction, and as an ontological description, the notion permits much intrinsic variation, meaning that a person does not have to think the same thoughts or engage in the same level of thought all the time.

If human personhood resides in a state of critical self-conscious awareness this may be 'as good as it gets', as there may not be a more complete definition. Personhood can be defined neither in biological nor in genetic terms. It cannot be the same as consciousness in that a person is still a person when unconscious, but that does not stop consciousness and personhood from being very closely linked. Personhood has nothing to do with the faculty of speech, with intellectual capacity or with any physical attributes, but it is about being human and having some sense of separate personal identity, especially (but not limited to) when it is self-consciously perceived.

Questions surrounding consciousness provide much fertile ground for discussion but will always remain troublesome when what is sought is irrefutable, concrete proof, and the problem of consciousness has been described as the last unanswered question in the history of philosophy, which points straight back to the question of metaphysics. This therefore provides a suitable point at which to close the chapter and move on to consider matters relating more specifically to clinical medicine and palliative care. In conclusion, understanding consciousness potentially enables one to understand more about persons and what it means to be a human being.[20] It also helps provide a better perspective for resolving some of the tension surrounding rights, including the right to expressions of personal autonomy in deciding on a course of treatment or other medical intervention.

Glossary of some useful ethical terms

casuistry – a method of assessing the morality of individual cases (e.g. those involving particular circumstances having certain defining characteristics)

consequentialism – stressing means above ends; ensuring a good outcome regardless of how it is achieved

deontology – the theory or study of rights and moral obligation

distributive justice – a practical expression of social justice (e.g. providing a method for the organisation and distribution of primary goods and services)

elenchus (sic elenchic) – (Gr.) literally a refutation, i.e. a type of philosophical argument or dialogue in the form of question and answer in which the teacher goes on to refute the opinions of a student

empiricism – a movement that has its origins in the seventeenth century concerned with the exploration (and defence of) scientifically derived knowledge; hence epistemic knowledge – that which is potentially capable of a measure of objective proof

epistemology (sic epistemic) – the study of that which concerns the nature of (scientific) knowledge

ethics – a branch of philosophy dating at least back to ancient Greece (e.g. the *Socratic Dialogues* of Plato or Aristotle's *Nicomachean Ethics*); the study of how we live with particular reference to (professional) standards of moral behaviour

hedonism – the pursuit of pleasure as an end in itself

metaphysics – the science of the fundamentals of all existence; a method of analysis not reliant upon applying rules of logic, neither limited to nor defined by reference to empirically driven knowledge

morals – the values by which people live; a synonym for *ethics*

normative – that which pertains to a norm or standard of conduct, i.e. defined by reference to usage more than general principle

ontology – the study of the science of being (i.e. what something is, not what it does or how it does it)

positivism – a theory that avoids metaphysical speculation (and natural law theory), giving priority to verifiable, empirically derived knowledge; *legal* positivism based on a premiss that the foundations of a legal system should be described in morally neutral terms; analysis of the role of law by reference to the society in which it operates

social justice – justice in society, characterised by criteria of social inclusion

teleology – a method of explanation or study that refers to ideas or events as being what they are 'by nature' in relation to 'the state of nature'

utility – a consequentialist method of reasoning, i.e. placing emphasis on ends rather than means; maximising happiness, affording it moral worth; a theory of justice stressing the greatest good for the greatest number of people

Dates of some prominent philosophers

Pythagoras	?570–?495 BCE
Socrates	469–399 BCE
Hippocrates	?460–?377 BCE
Plato	427–347 BCE
Aristotle	384–322 BCE
Galen	129–215 CE
Aquinas	1225–1274
Galilei	1564–1642
Hobbes	1588–1679
Gassendi	1592–1655
Descartes	1596–1650
Boyle	1627–1691
Spinoza	1632–1677
Locke	1632–1704
Newton	1642–1727
Leibnitz	1646–1716
Berkeley	1685–1753
Hume	1711–1776
Rousseau	1712–1788
Kant	1724–1804
Bentham	1748–1832
Hegel	1770–1831
Austin	1790–1859
Mill	1806–1873
Sidgwick	1838–1900
James W	1842–1910
Nietzsche	1844–1900
Royce	1855–1916
Husserl	1859–1938
Dewey	1859–1952
Whitehead	1861–1947
Russell	1872–1970
Moore GE	1873–1958
Wittgenstein	1889–1951
Heidegger	1889–1976
Tarski	1902–1983
Popper	1902–1994
Hart HLA	1907–1992
Rawls	1921–2002
Dworkin R	1931–
Nozick	1938–2002

Notes to Chapter 2

1. Cf. Yu J (2003).
2. See glossary of terms.
3. Plato *Apologia* 38a (Vlastos, 1980).
4. Therefore, genotypical characteristics may be considered teleological, but phenotypical characteristics *not,* even though the analogy should not be stretched too far.
5. Thomas Aquinas was an able Aristotelian scholar, but as a clergyman his philosophy sometimes put him in open conflict with his theology. Philosophical speculation was not without attendant risks, especially in the light of the historical powers of the church as an institution.
6. Cf. White (1997).
7. Ideally, mind should be described without using the definite article as a prefix (i.e. as a generic term describing a universal not a particular, whereby mind is a principle that works *through* the vehicle of the brain), but this notion is contentious in relation to Western analytic philosophy, having its origin in Classical Indian philosophy.
8. A chunk of eighteenth-century philosophical history has been omitted here, which would have included the Scottish moral philosopher David Hume (among others), had chronology been an organising theme for the chapter.
9. See the glossary on page 24 for an explanation of technical philosophical terms.
10. Sen *Equality of What?* in Rawls (1987).
11. Cf. the scenarios in Part Two.
12. Kegley *Community, Autonomy and Managed Care,* quoted in McGee (2003) *Pragmatic Bioethics* (2e).
13. Mill (1860) *On Liberty* (Chapter 4).
14. Hart (2001: Chapter 3) writes on late twentieth-century disparities between American deontological social values and English utilitarian social values.
15. Williams B A critique of utilitarianism In: Smart and Williams (1973).
16. *See* Chapter 3 for further discussion on this topic.
17. Coleman (2001: Lectures 11 and 12) in which Coleman writes about the Rule of Recognition which 'comes into existence as a rule that regulates behaviour only if it is *practised*'. However, according to the Social Fact Thesis, 'the grounds of the criteria of legality in every community that has law are [to be regarded as] a matter of social fact'.
18. The question of autonomy and rights is dealt with more fully in Chapter 5.
19. Although health is not directly addressed in the Human Rights Act 1998, some articles have potential applications (*see* Chapter 5).
20. Cf. Worthington (2002) for more detailed analysis of the whole question of consciousness.

Chapter 3

Critical decisions: moving from theory to practice

Models of decision making

The conceptual basis for making difficult decisions is an interesting topic, and is worthy of separate study. In the context of applied ethics, careful analysis is needed in order to be able to identify the basis upon which critical decisions are made. Theories of decision making vary greatly, and they encompass several domains ranging from multi-professionalism, logic and democratic justice, to game theory, principleism and the philosophy of law. When the issues in question concern matters of life and death and personal values and choice, as in the case of ethics in palliative care, they demand serious attention. Some potentially useful models are considered below in order to assess if and how they work in clinical settings in general, and in end-of-life situations in particular. In the terms of making ethical decisions it would be harbouring an illusion to suppose that there were going to be definitively right or wrong answers to particular problems. 'Most appropriate' or 'least worst' would be better terms to use than 'right' or 'wrong' in ethical deliberations. It is not the intention to consider the ethics just in terms of black and white or to view it in isolation. The intention instead is to consider theoretical models and processes of decision making, which include but are not limited to ethics, and to assess their applicability in the clinical setting.[1]

Multi-professionalism and team decisions

The extent to which multi-professionalism is a practical reality depends on the setting within which decisions are made, and there is no reason why multi-professionalism should necessarily be afforded equal importance in all the different specialty areas of medicine. The desirability of multi-professionalism as an approach to critical decision making is clear insofar as potentially each member of a team has something useful to contribute. While different specialties work in different ways, clinical oncology and palliative care present themselves as natural candidates in which clinicians can work as part of a multi-professional team.

Accepting that limitations exist in relation to all models of reasoning, there is evidence in favour of endorsing the concept of multi-professionalism. According to the Higher Education Funding Council for England, reasons for encouraging multi-professionalism in medical training are 'so that doctors, nurses and other health professionals can work more effectively together'.[2] Theoretically, a multi-professional team ought to be capable of reaching a balanced decision, and to benefit from the synergy arising from interaction between various members of the team. However, it cannot just be assumed that everyone believes in the benefits of team decision making or considers themselves an effective team player, so when it comes to turning theory into practice the aims and objectives of multi-professionalism cannot be taken for granted.

The evidence base used in decision making is quite logically linked to particular specialty areas, but partly because of a continuing trend towards specialisation and sub-specialisation, the evidence base may not concern itself with more broadly based patient concerns. While the need for empirical evidence relating to each patient and each clinical situation is not in dispute, this does not preclude the need for additional information being made available to help provide a more complete profile of each patient. This means there should be recognition of the fact that a patient is more than just a collection of symptoms. It is too easy to label patients according to their primary complaint, while leaving secondary complaints to other specialists and leaving the person out of the picture altogether. Multi-professionalism ought to help promote a greater responsiveness to the needs of individual patients as persons.

In an era of targets and outcomes, frequently measured according to economic units of treatment, it can present difficulty evaluating a patient as more than just someone with a particular medical condition. This may be the fault of the individual clinician who sees no need to form an holistic judgment, but equally likely it is the fault of systems that lack flexibility and that have to record data according to categories, filling in tick-boxes on a screen. This points in the direction of an increasingly important role for multi-professional teams to try and help counter the fragmentation of delivering unco-ordinated episodes of care.[3]

With teams, it is not just the diverse nature of information provided that is potentially valuable, but also the nature and quality of the interaction between team members. If employed effectively, multi-professional teams can build a broad profile of an individual patient and help reduce the risk of error arising from a failure to communicate or a failure to cross-reference and locate data stored on different systems.[4] Furthermore, where appropriate, interaction can even extend beyond clinical team members to include family members as well, some of whom can have a major role to play in terms of helping inform decisions made by the multi-professional team. Family members do not attend ward rounds but if their views are known they can at least be taken into consideration when key decisions are made. The benefits to be gained from the adoption of a broad matrix for making critical decisions and consulting with major stakeholders in each different case may be considerable, even though such benefits are not easy to quantify.

Teams are likely to arrive at decisions via routes that differ from those taken by individuals working alone. Thus, not only is it important to pool expertise, but it is also important to evaluate the team decision-making process itself. If effectively employed it can help counterbalance personal, clinical judgments formulated from a narrowly defined base of evidence. Within the palliative care setting benefits should indeed be gained from team building and shared decision making, and there would seem to be far greater risks associated with *not* adopting such methods than with multi-professionalism being adopted and incorporated into regular clinical use.

Logical analysis

Logical analysis has relevance both in the multi-professional team setting and in the context of deliberation by individual clinicians. Although logic often uses hypotheses, formulae and the construction of arguments about truth-claims, it does not mean that all forms of logic work in the same way. Logical analysis can be applied as a method of reasoning that can be of help in arriving at a point where a claim can be made such that other possibilities can safely be excluded from consideration. It can potentially allow for a firm conclusion to be reached to a particular problem by eliminating solutions that do not work, thus making it easier to focus on those that do. In that decision-making skills are indeed capable of analysis, methods used need not be a matter of mystique. Such knowledge can be deliberately acquired even if, clinically speaking, the processes are not often subject to regular scrutiny.

Arguments are sometimes constructed in philosophy using expressions such as 'if this, then that' or 'if this material fact does not apply to a particular case, then that points to a conclusion such that proposition '*P*' cannot be the case'. It is not necessary here for such expressions to be given a label, but, if considered as part of a method of reasoning, it becomes easier to balance one proposition against another by systematically assembling known facts and making provision for facts that are still unknown. This can be a valid way of performing differential diagnosis, and of evaluating the balance of probabilities to a point where a particular outcome for a patient can be said to be desirable and/or achievable.

At an informal level this method of analysis can reliably inform clinical reasoning by fulfilling criteria for sharp and clear use of language, and by using reasoning skills that can be demonstrated to colleagues involved in the management of a particular case. Logical analysis can assume various different forms (e.g. using either inductive or deductive methods of reasoning); Russell (1938) went so far as to say that 'mathematics and logic are identical', but that is perhaps going too far. In practical terms it is not the establishment of irrefutable proof of an argument or line of reasoning that is necessarily the main aim. Rather it is the *process* of reasoning that assumes particular importance, and this can well be developed into a system of argumentation.

Argumentation is a chain of reasoning whereby it is not so much the outcome of a decision that matters as the method and process by which it came about, which typically applies in cases involving complex ethical analysis. In clinical scenarios there are often several different strands to an argument (e.g. relating to the patient's circumstances and the patient's family as well as clinical matters relating to physical signs and symptoms). These have to be woven together in order to try and arrive at a decision, and such a process is especially valuable in relation to patients who are incapacitated or otherwise unable to take an active part in arriving at a final decision on the best way to proceed. In other situations, logical analysis can be employed in helping determine the best options to put forward to a patient. Although in some cases there may be few viable alternatives, as could be the case in managing an end-stage cancer, at other times, for example when diagnosis and prognosis are still uncertain, logical analysis could be utilised (directly or indirectly) to good effect.

Democratic justice

In terms of other theories, in the political arena democracy is upheld as the gold standard for making collective decisions. There may be other applications for democratic theory as well, but the extent to which democratic justice provides a workable model for decision making in the clinical arena is very much influenced by hierarchical structures that exist within medicine.[5] Although these may be less conspicuous than a quarter of a century ago when medical decision making was much more autocratic, there are issues that still need to be resolved before democratic principles can readily find their way into the hospital. General respect for notions of accountability and justice is not in question, but it remains to be seen how well justice and democracy can be applied in a clinical setting.

Many of the values associated with modern liberal democracies are founded on notions for which there is no meta-theory that can provide an accurate, comprehensive account, and that includes democracy.[6] If principles of democracy and justice succeed in providing an effective clinical model for making decisions, their use would be indicative of a step in the direction away from medical paternalism. Democratic justice, however, is not the engine that provides the driving force away from medical paternalism. That comes from respect for patient autonomy, and respect for the rights of the individual to decide what s/he wants done or not done, which has a quite different focus. Democratic decision making has a collective focus, whereas rights to autonomy are directed towards the individual, and so they pull in the opposite direction. But if instead democratic justice is substituted for multi-professional team decision making then the situation appears quite different. The main difficulty here is over how to proceed from a theoretical to an applied base in terms of finding the most effective model for collective decisions.

Democratic choice in medicine is not a subject that is often addressed directly, any more than democratic justice finds its way on to medical conference agendas, unless, that is, it is focused on a topic such as access to healthcare or the ethics of distribution. Applied democratic values have clear relevance in the healthcare setting in the context of fairness, equity, access to services and the distribution of scarce resources. But clinical decisions affecting the care of individuals will probably only be addressed in this way in the event of a challenge to policy decisions, such as a decision not to fund a specific form of treatment.

Democratic principles and majority voting can be subject to differences in interpretation and analysis by different political scientists,[7] but nonetheless, it would be unwise to dismiss the principle too hastily. Collective decision making does not automatically imply that all parties to a decision have an equal voice. In a clinical management model, equal voting is less important than active participation in the decision-making process, and the demonstration of respect for differences in personal values and beliefs. Therefore, in the clinical environment, respect for persons is generally a more useful concept than equality of representation. Head counting is a crude method to use to formulate clinical decisions; furthermore, as has long been known, if the number of participants in an exercise in democratic choice is small, then it becomes mathematically unreliable to use such an expression of choice as a method for reaching a decision.[8] Therefore, on balance, this method of decision making has its place even if not in an everyday clinical scenario.

Game theory

Another topic worth discussing is game theory, and by way of explanation it has been said that:

> Game theory is the most important and useful tool in the analyst's kit whenever she confronts situations in which one agent's rational decision making depends on her expectations about what one or more other agents will do, and theirs similarly depend on expectations about her (Ross, 2002).

But while game theory pertains to the interaction between different parties to a decision, in the clinical setting, significant limitations apply. First, it is more normal for it to be applied in the context of economic decision making. Second, there is no provision for key players being unable to participate in the process, and so it could not be applied in relation to non-competent patients, and third, it is not clear whether game theory can be adapted to reflect the doctor–patient relationship. It may be that it is more applicable to decisions made between clinicians than between clinician and patient.

While a patient might answer a question in such a way as to second guess what the response might be from a clinician, modifying the answer in order to try and achieve a desired personal outcome or goal, this would be different from exercising personal autonomy – it would be about employing a strategy in which key players (e.g. patient and doctor) modified their behaviour so as to avoid confronting unwanted facts or eliciting an unsatisfactory response. Even if such games were played out at the bedside or in the consulting room that would not give them ethical validity, and neither would it mean they could be upheld as a viable model.

Game theory is a mixture of mathematics and psychology, and it could provide a model for planning health strategy, and it could conceivably be of help in facilitating a team decision. Psychology certainly plays a part in how interactions work between different members of a team; furthermore, economics already play a part in setting the parameters within which clinical decisions often have to be made (especially where politically driven policies impinge on the practice of clinical medicine). However, games and numbers are not the favoured option when it comes to finding the most effective model for making ethical evaluations in difficult cases. Once again, this application may be more suited to the policy environment than to the practical delivery of individual episodes of care.

Principleism

Presently, most clinical models for resolving ethical dilemmas defer to the four 'classic' bioethical principles of autonomy, beneficence, non-maleficence and justice. These were discussed in the previous chapter, but it is worth giving further consideration to the usefulness of this method, in spite of it being subject to inherent limitations. These partly arise from reliance upon abstract concepts that do not sit well with scientifically derived clinical evidence. Such concepts have the tendency to give rise to questions that lead to further questions, or else to defer to absolute moral principles about which there is little or no agreement. The four principles provide a basic taxonomy of ethical categories with which some clinicians may already be familiar, but nonetheless, their validity is unproven in the context of applied medical ethics and making critical decisions. Being used does not give a method validity on its own; that is measured in terms of how well a given method achieves its aim, which is not the same thing.

It was originally intended for 'the four principles' to provide benchmark reference points for use when assessing the merits and demerits of cases that presented clinicians with an ethical dilemma.[9] However, the reality is that these points are not points at all but broad categories presenting in the form of abstract moral principles. Individual components of a clinical case coming together and presenting parties to a decision with an ethical dilemma are, first, unlikely to sit neatly within a single category and, second, if different components pertain to different categories they can easily be in conflict one with another, hence of limited use in trying to find a practical solution. It is too inhibiting to limit the scope of reasoning by trying to relate the facts of a case to one or more of the principles; that process can be restricting and have quite the opposite effect of opening up thinking to the consideration of all available options. As a model for decision making it does not appear to stand up well to critical analysis.

Legal theory

It is time now to consider decisions made within the context of law and its theoretical underpinning. Legal decisions do not employ any one uniform model of reasoning – that has to be a matter for legal practitioners and individual judges to decide. However, as with other models, there is a question of whether and how jurisprudential reasoning has practical relevance within the context of medical decision making. Some philosophical aspects of the role of law were referred to in the previous chapter, and the relationship between legality and morality feature in the next chapter in the context of decisions about assisted death. So given this recurring theme, it should be clear by this stage that a case is being made to the effect that jurisprudence can be employed to good effect for the present purposes. In particular, it can be effectively interwoven with the thread of medical ethics in general, as well as with ethics at the end of life.[10]

The basis of the relationship between law and morals, consciously or otherwise, influences the nature of the discourse between lawyers, philosophers, lawmakers and practising clinicians. This cannot be taken to infer that law and morals are different expressions of the same thing, or that law is based on nothing more than common-sense morality, or that moral standards can be defined only in relation to what is or is not lawful. Such assumptions fail to capture the essence of the relationship between law and morality and in particular, they overlook important aspects of law that relate to society and how law functions at the social level. But accepting that there is a dynamic relationship between them both avoids the pitfall of having to defer to absolute moral principles, and avoids reliance on the assumption that for something to be lawful it will necessarily also be moral, or that for something to be moral it will necessarily be lawful.

By being broadly based, a set of rules that is conceptually clear, socially inclusive and devoid of wrongful discrimination is indicative of a fair and reasonable basis upon which law can reliably function. As an ethical position, this type of jurisprudential reasoning encourages social diversity, and its inclusivity can favour practical applications such as might occur in a clinical setting. More work needs to be done before the viability of this method can be established 'beyond reasonable doubt', but it is indicative of a promising and useful avenue down which to try and travel.

As a branch of moral philosophy, jurisprudence is capable of scientific modes of application without compromising its ability to help form evaluative judgments. It can be sharp and analytical, and at the same time it can be utilised in a way that it is sensitive to social and moral concerns. Accepting the limitation that jurisprudence itself is not easy to define, and that its language may be inaccessible to those without special knowledge, at a theoretical level it is offered as the method of choice when it comes to informing critical decision making and trying to resolve ethical dilemmas. It has greater relevance than other models, and it does not rely on the application of morally blind formulae. Furthermore, it encompasses and is not separate from logical analysis, and logical analysis is itself frequently employed in practical jurisprudence.

Legal theory provides a tool that can help in trying to arrive at critical decisions in a way that is fair, rational, and capable of taking into account all relevant information, be it social, moral or medical in nature. None of the other models reviewed has this combination of attributes. Granted, it cannot just be picked up and utilised without being the subject of further scrutiny, and a process still has to be identified that would more easily facilitate the move from theory to practice. But what analytic jurisprudence can do is offer a reliable tool for critical reasoning that can be used to underpin more practical modes of application.

Roles and responsibilities

English law is quite specific about who is allowed to decide what and for whom, and in the case of the non-competent adult no one is allowed to consent on his or her behalf.[11] Clinicians alone have to decide on appropriate action on the basis of what is likely to be in the person's best interests. But it has to be remembered that however incapacitated a patient might be, that patient remains a person up to and including the moment of death and should be treated accordingly with due respect. Currently that may not always be the case, and it is a circular argument to try and define best interests by reference to what is essentially a subjective standard. It also presupposes that what is best for one person is probably best for another person similarly placed, which should not just be assumed.[12] Overall, it is to be welcomed that these matters are currently under review as regards the law in England and Wales.[13]

Increasingly, where time allows and where the courts are not involved, difficult decisions are put before a clinical ethics committee. However, the role of clinical ethics committees is not clearly defined, being a quite recent introduction to the UK.[14] Committees can debate the relative merits of a case and identify key issues without necessarily arriving at a definite conclusion, and so they should not be relied upon to indicate a way forward in difficult cases. At the present stage of things, with the format and workings of clinical ethics committees still very much evolving, no unified model has been established that defines how they operate, who their members are, and if and how committee members are specially trained.[15]

Questions of equilibrium

One thing that has not been discussed so far is establishing equilibrium within the process of deliberation. The term 'equilibrium' is employed to refer to a state in which internal forces are held in balance one with another. Such a state may be helpful in guarding against power imbalances that can distort values attaching to different points of view. Furthermore, establishing equilibrium can help avoid extremes of viewpoint that militate against reaching balanced, rational, collective decisions. Thus far everything is positive, but as a hypothetical position it may not fit within the broader premiss of applied ethics, by reason of making insufficient allowance for the expression of personal values that can easily upset the equilibrium and militate against the likelihood of achieving a resolution in cases where there is strong disagreement.

Were all forces to be held in perfect balance, which would be a true equilibrium,[16] it could be more difficult not less difficult for parties to a decision to identify and then agree upon a particular course of action. On the face of it, if in an ideal state all parties were to hold an equal share of power, demonstrating mutual respect for each other's views, then it would seem acceptable for that to form the basis of a collective decision. However, in practice it cannot work for two reasons. First, medicine is hierarchical in the way it operates and where team decisions are made, there is someone in overall charge whose responsibility it is to defend decisions if they are subsequently challenged. Second, it does not allow for the expression of patient autonomy (i.e. the right of a competent patient to accept or refuse a medical treatment or intervention, irrespective of how many people thought it was a good or bad idea). Thus, with competent patients, power is titled towards the patient and away from the practising clinician, and with patients lacking capacity the reverse is likely to apply. Therefore, decisions made by striving to arrive at a stable equilibrium within the decision-making matrix could be unworkable, or even unethical if other considerations, such as the moral value of self-directed medical decision making (now widely accepted as the legal standard), come to be overlooked.

Discussion points

When searching for a workable solution to questions about protocol and models of decision making, there clearly needs to be a measure of adaptation in order to facilitate the potentially difficult translation from theory to practice. For example, the most refined model for decision making may be insufficiently patient centred to be of value in the hospital setting. What may be needed instead is a different type of equilibrium in which all key stakeholders participate while still recognising that, wherever possible, patient choice takes precedence.

Weighing risks and benefits is an integral part of the calculus of arriving at an informed decision as regards a proposed medical intervention, and in the context of making ethically sound clinical decisions the following points may need to be considered:

- risks of harm (including variables relating to the probability, frequency and severity of various harms) and the likelihood or not of achieving a desired outcome
- genuine uncertainty about a course of action on the part of a patient, a patient's family and/or the clinical team
- wishes of the next of kin being different from the wishes of other members of the family, or an advance directive being applicable to a given situation but indicating a course of action contrary to everyone else's feelings and intuitions
- cultural or religious values and beliefs held by a patient and/or a patient's family indicating a course of action in opposition to clinically held beliefs and opinions.

It would be naïve to suppose that with these potential complications there is ever going to be an easy route to follow. But the effort has to be worth making, especially when so much now rides on the validity of patient consent. The intention here is to try and identify a method of reasoning that is most likely to avoid or resolve conflicts. Central to the entire process is the respect that needs to be shown to the rights and needs of patients as persons. But it is also fair to suppose that benefits accrue to all those involved in decision making if the process itself is better understood.

As a working conclusion, the decision-making process is best viewed as a collective one, while recognising that patient wishes are always paramount. The process should be as fair and inclusive as is practically possible; it should be capable of standing up to critical reasoned argument, while avoiding unnecessary secrecy. Ethical reasoning (especially that which is based on jurisprudential analysis) is potentially capable of fulfilling the criteria for making reasoned and informed decisions in a way that is fully integrated with clinically-derived criteria. In the final analysis, bad ethics is no different from bad science – both fail to live up to their ideals and achieve their true potential. But there is no reason why 'good ethics' cannot coexist alongside 'good science', and where properly executed in the clinical arena, good ethics and good science should not be in conflict with each other. In the transition from theory to practice, careful consideration therefore needs to be given to all factors involved in making sound clinical decisions.

Notes to Chapter 3

[1] For an alternative version of this chapter, with information on ethical frameworks and methods of seeking informed patient consent, see Webb P (2005) *Ethical Issues in Palliative Care* (2e). Radcliffe Publishing, Oxford. Chapter 2).

[2] Higher Education Funding Council for England press release, 30 March 2001: www.hefce.ac.uk/news/HEFCE/2001/medical.htm.

[3] The composition of a multi-professional team working in the hospital setting will vary according to the type of setting, and the type of care being planned. In the NHS the ward round provides the most obvious example of multi-professional teams at work.

This kind of team could comprise a senior consultant, other consultants who may be on duty, senior house officers and specialist registrars, senior members of the nursing team, and any key allied health professionals.

4 Cf. Rowe M (2004) Doctors' responses to medical errors. *Crit Rev Oncol/Hematol.* **52:** 147–63.

5 The relationship between hierarchical power structures and the exercise of democracy is not something that can be properly discussed here, but they are not mutually exclusive concepts. The way in which hierarchical power structures and democratic justice interrelate is far from clear (e.g. in established institutions and social structures)

6 Cf. Shapiro I (1999) *Democratic Justice.* Yale University Press, Connecticut. Chapter 5.

7 *Ibid.*

8 There is a body of social choice literature on this topic that dates back to Marquis de Condorcet's famous *Essay on the Application of Analysis to the Probability of Decisions Reached by a Majority of Votes (1785).* For recent literature on the topic see works by Schumpeter JA, Waldron J, Goodin R, Young P, Coleman J, Arrow KJ, and others.

9 Beauchamp TL and Childress JF (1979) *Biomedical Ethics.* Oxford University Press, Oxford.

10 The term jurisprudence is used here to refer to formal analysis about the content and nature of law. This is something separate from the body of law and its methods of implementation, and it reflects the way that law is actually practised in society.

11 Pending a change in the law – see below.

12 Cf. Worthington (2002) Clinical issues on consent: some philosophical concerns *J Med Eth.* **28**: 377–80.

13 Cf. *Mental Capacity Bill* (2004), at the committee stage in the House of Lords at the time of going to press, and Cf. Draft Code of Practice for Mental Capacity Bill: www.dca.gov.uk/menincap/legis.htm.

14 Clinical ethics committees have long been in use in the USA, but because the model of healthcare delivery is so different from that in the UK, a process of adaptation is needed before such committees can be imported into routine use within the NHS.

15 Cf. UK Clinical Ethics Network for further information on the role and function of clinical ethics committees: www.ethics-network.org.uk.

16 Cf. Skyrms B (1996) *Evolution of the Social Contract.* Cambridge University Press, Cambridge.

Chapter 4

Decisions at the end of life

Autonomy and the use of advance statements

Following on from the more theoretical discussions of the last chapter, some important moral and legal issues concerning end-of-life decisions need to be addressed in the context of applied ethics. Arguments surrounding advance statements, euthanasia and requests for assistance in bringing life to an end are to be discussed, as well as well-known topics such as killing and letting die, and the use of 'do not attempt resuscitation' decisions. Discussion takes place within a broad context of moral and legal discourse, and while it is understood that autonomy is a basic right that competent adults deserve to have respected, questions arise in terms of how far it extends in end-of-life situations. The basis of advance statements centres around the rights of individual patients, and although overall autonomy is key in terms of law and ethics, it may not be indicative of practical solutions, especially when applied as an absolute moral principle.

The right to make advance statements may soon pass into law in England and Wales via the Mental Capacity Bill (2004). This follows on from the example set by the Adults with Incapacity Act (Scotland) 2000, and it should bring England and Wales more into line with the rest of Europe. The Bill uses the term 'advance statements' as opposed to 'advance directives'; this is ontologically sound in that an incapacitated patient cannot direct clinicians to do (or not to do) very much, but anyone can express what they would or would not like done should a particular medical situation arise. The patient makes a statement of wishes and intentions based not on presenting facts, which are unknown, but on personal beliefs and values; these wishes should, where possible, be respected. In reality, things are not always simple and it is not possible to antic-ipate either what might happen at some point in the future or what one might feel at the time. One cannot readily project a psychological state into the future, and while a mindset may be anticipated based on personal beliefs and prefer-ences, the mind state of a patient at a particular point in time may be totally different.

Family members may have opposing views amongst themselves, especially in a time of crisis, and there is ample scope for differing viewpoints to come to the fore when a patient loses decision-making capacity. However, for the capacitous patient the desire to hold on to life is usually very strong, and it may over-ride previous intentions of wanting to refuse active treatment and have life-sustain-ing treatment (such as artificial feeding and hydration) terminated.[1] In other words, if any degree of capacity is retained, one needs to be allowed to change one's mind as a situation develops. It is inadvisable to be overly prescriptive in trying to direct those charged with looking after one's future general medical needs; however, where a patient is diagnosed as suffering from a degenerative, progressive disease like Alzheimer's that results in eventual loss of capacity, the situation may be different. It would then be reasonable to indicate, even in unambiguous terms, what one's wishes might then be in the belief that those wishes would be respected. While patients do not have a right to demand any particular intervention, making an advance statement constitutes an expression of autonomy that can provide safeguards against well-intentioned but possibly misinformed judgments made by others.[2]

It has to be remembered that an advance statement has only limited power to influence what happens in 'real time', however well it is drafted. In particular, it cannot force a clinician to do anything that is contrary to the law. The key to understanding how advance statements ought to work is in an appreciation of the difference between clinically indicated patient need, in which the clinician forms an assessment and makes a decision based on knowledge of similar cases, and value-based decisions made by the patient, which have different criteria from those based on medical needs alone. An advance statement is designed to protect the beliefs and desires of someone unable to express contemporaneous wishes. Such wishes may coincide with a course of action that is clinically indicated – but they may not, which can give rise to tension, and advance statements are not always popular with clinicians.

In order for advance statements to be effective, mechanisms have to be in place for the service provider to know whether, on admission to hospital, a patient has made a valid and relevant prior statement and if so, what it contains.[3] Furthermore, a system of administration must allow for the appointment of a health proxy, i.e. someone charged with lasting power of (medical) attorney to act as an appointed representative to look after the personal best interests of the patient after capacity has been lost.[4] Advance statements are relatively ineffective without this facility, but it should be recognised that the role of health proxy may be a difficult one to fulfil and is not one to be undertaken lightly. It is of little use appointing a proxy decision-maker if the person appointed does not know anything about the patient's wishes or, for that matter, is him/herself rather indecisive in nature. Great care should be taken before conferring this degree of responsibility on to another person. While a proxy may hold personal views opposed to those of the patient, this need not matter provided that there is a clear understanding between a would-be patient and her proxy.

A special court, called the Court of Protection, will be constituted to appoint a representative through the office of the Public Guardian to look after the interests of non-competent patients who have no one acting on their behalf.[5] While it remains to be seen how well these arrangements will work in practice, their introduction should amount to a significant improvement over current arrangements with regard to the limited rights of patients lacking capacity. Making this step provides positive re-inforcement for the rights of patients as persons, and for anyone losing the ability to exercise the right to autonomy. In short, respect for persons extends further than respect for autonomy; the latter can be lost through accident or injury and is subject to inherent limitations; the former extends all the way to the time of death and is without precondition. Autonomy can be lost and regained whereas personhood is invariant, and this distinction is worth bearing in mind.

Euthanasia and assisted suicide

There is often confusion of terminology with respect to different categories of euthanasia, and it will be as well to try and clear this up. Assisted suicide (by physician or others) is a type of euthanasia but key differences exist concerning who performs the act. Assisted suicide is just that – it is an act carried out by the patient but with the help of others; euthanasia, on the other hand, is generally performed by someone other than the patient. The term euthanasia simply means 'good death', 'eu' meaning happy and 'thanatos' meaning death, although it is widely interpreted as meaning 'mercy killing' and hence involving someone else. While it would be futile to challenge commonly accepted usage, it should be remembered that so-called mercy killing is only based on a loose interpretation of the original Greek.

If the act of euthanasia is carried out by the patient without external assistance it is an act of suicide, hence legal and protected by Parliament under the terms of the Suicide Act 1961. However, it remains illegal to assist someone else in this act, and when a physician is called upon to lend assistance in providing the means to enable a patient to end his/her own life, it is described as 'physician-assisted suicide' (PAS). PAS is illegal throughout the UK and is only legal in certain parts of the world.[6]

The various types of euthanasia are as follows:

- voluntary
- involuntary
- active
- passive.

Voluntary euthanasia is that which is requested by the patient in accord with an express or determined wish.

Involuntary euthanasia is an act of killing, certainly if it is against the wishes of a patient. However, there is no clear agreement about what is covered under this term.[7]

Active euthanasia can be voluntary or involuntary; PAS generally falls under the category of being both active and voluntary. By contrast, involuntary but active euthanasia is murder plain and simple, permitting no justification or moral ambiguity. Involuntary active euthanasia is deliberate killing without either a patient's consent or active participation (as in the case of Harold Shipman, the Manchester GP convicted in 2000 of multiple murder after deliberately killing large numbers of patients under his care).[8]

Passive euthanasia in the literal sense need not be euthanasia at all. Passive euthanasia may be the result of either an act or an omission, and it may be either voluntary or involuntary. Withholding or withdrawing treatment can fall under this heading in cases where a patient is effectively allowed to die from an underlying medical condition. When a decision is made on whether or not to continue, start or cease medical intervention, difficulties can arise and this is where clinical guidelines may need to be consulted.[9] Withholding treatment is legitimate if further treatment is unlikely to produce any significant benefit and only result in further unnecessary suffering; however, withdrawing treatment already begun is sometimes more complicated and can necessitate obtaining a court order (e.g. in cases of persistent or permanent vegetative state – a form of irreversible coma).[10]

Given the above it would be an oversimplification to suggest that all forms of euthanasia should be either banned or made legal.[11] In reality, where euthanasia is legal it is not all forms that come under the heading of permissibility, and those categories that are permitted are generally covered by strict codes of conduct.[12] The Dutch law (2002)[13] is perhaps the most liberal of all and was designed to remove the threat of legal sanctions, even though in reality none had previously been imposed for many years. Now that it is regulated, it would appear that not all clinicians follow the letter of the law in terms of adhering to the protocols (Sheldon, 2004). Legislation does not always act in the way that it is first intended, and in the Netherlands it may be more difficult than before to compile accurate data on causes of death and the role played by clinicians at or around the time of death.

What the 'for and against euthanasia' arguments bring sharply into focus is the primary role of the physician and attitudes of society towards death and dying and the care of the terminally ill.[14] There is little evidence to suggest that legalising PAS opens the door to its widespread use. In the state of Oregon, for instance, numbers of patients choosing this option and following through with the act represent only a tiny proportion of terminally ill patients. Slippery slopes do not always become manifest, and allowing some forms of assisted suicide does not mean that other forms of euthanasia necessarily follow suit in terms of permissibility, or that options available under the law will be actively sought by ever-increasing numbers of patients. Advocates for euthanasia argue that individual rights should trump all other considerations, and that everyone should have the maximum say in determining the time and manner of death as an ultimate expression of autonomy. But on the other side of the argument, those who are against tend to argue that causing death is intrinsically wrong, however it is controlled or brought about. This could arise from adherence to a Kantian ethic, based on moral imperatives and the inviolability of the human body; it could be based on formal religious objections. Then again, arguments against euthanasia could be derived from a utilitarian ethic such that causing or assisting in causing death never maximises general well-being, and removing the burden of a severely ill patient does not in any way benefit the community as whole.

Finally, it can be argued that deliberately causing or hastening the death of a patient is a perversion of the fundamental duties of a doctor, and in direct opposition to the Hippocratic Oath and modern codes of best practice. This comprises a fairly powerful argument, especially if personal objections are factored in, and anyone debating this issue will need to weigh these arguments and see which ones speak to them most clearly. There is no shortage of literature on the topic, and merely performing a keyword search on the Internet will reveal a whole range of views from different protagonists on either side of the debate. For instance, journals such as the *New England Journal of Medicine* do carry full-length articles on the topic from time to time.[15]

Interestingly, questions arise relating to this topic about whether changing the law to accommodate the views of society or a section of the public that, for instance, supports PAS thereby makes it moral or that leaving most forms of euthanasia outside the law (as in the UK) ensures that the act itself remains immoral.[16] This brings us back to the point where the potential difference between being legal and being moral needs to be explored further.

Morality and legality (revisited)[17]

Arguments about the difference between what is ethical, what is legal and what is both (or neither) can leave readers with just a passing interest in such things either irritated or bemused. Furthermore, clinicians sometimes express frustration that reading the literature on law and morality only gives rise to a list of unanswerable questions and hypothetical distinctions, and there can be an element of truth to this claim. But arguments about killing and letting die, for instance, address important issues and much can depend on how matters are interpreted, including whether or not it can be either moral or legal to hasten the death of another human being.

Moral distinctions are often cited in legal judgments,[18] but it is rash to assume that law is implicitly derived from a sense of public morals. The relationship between law and morals is discussed elsewhere (*see* Chapters 2 and 3), and there is a large quantity of scholarly work covering all different aspects of analytic jurisprudence that is independent of discourse about medical ethics in general.[19] However, it is maintained that as a method of reasoning analytic jurisprudence can provide a firm foundation for ethical reasoning. It is under-utilised in clinical ethics, perhaps for no other reason than that it appears inaccessible, but that need not be the case. As was argued in the previous chapter, potentially it has a key role to play in end-of-life decision making.

Moral values are things which can and should be respected, and upholding the rule of law is generally conducive to social stability and the well-being of the community. But individual members of society can have their own independent sense of morality, and members of society are not generally left to choose which laws to accept and which to ignore. Morality and legality are not always the same, and the discussion is not just about law and ethics. Intrinsically it is a three-way discussion about law, morality and society,[20] and it is time now to consider where this leads in terms of clinical cases and how they can be satisfactorily resolved according to the law and the social expression of morality.

Killing and letting die, acts and omissions, and withholding and withdrawing treatment

These distinctions can be crucial when making end-of-life decisions and, for example, doing nothing to intervene when a useful intervention could otherwise be made would at the very least be an act of negligence.[21] Omissions are not in themselves wrong; it depends on why an omission is made and what motivation is behind a decision not to intervene. Negligent action or inaction is defined according to legal criteria, and in order for negligence to be established the law requires that:

1 a position of trust must be found to exist between the clinician and patient that gives rise to a duty of care
2 the actions of the clinician fall short of what would thereby reasonably be expected and
3 actual harm ensued as a consequence of an act having not been done, or having been done badly to the clear detriment of the patient.

It could well be that an action causes harm from the unforeseen complications of a clinical intervention. Harm can arise as a result of errors in clinical judgment or the execution of a task, but this does not make the harm unlawful. Action that results in harm may well be unethical or unlawful, but each act or sequence of acts needs to be assessed according to its merits and so nothing can be presupposed. Medical harm, medical error and clinical negligence each have different definitions; on occasions they could coincide but these legal distinctions do not need to be addressed here.

Sometimes, where a patient dies as a result of action (or inaction), it can give rise to criminal investigations, in which case the distinction between killing and letting die could well come into play. Killing is essentially a positive act but killing can also happen indirectly by means of inaction, such as failing to respond in a medical emergency situation. Killing and letting die, and acts and omissions are two separate but linked distinctions and they should not be confused by supposing that killing is always the result of an act or that letting die is necessarily the result of some kind of omission. Certainly, killing as a wilful act is unlawful and contrary to accepted codes of medical practice but lines cannot always be sharply drawn.

Consider, for instance, where a patient is being kept alive on a ventilator. If the patient being ventilated is conscious and in possession of full legal capacity, then terminating necessary and wanted treatment could be a deliberate act of killing. But should a patient express the autonomous wish that she does not want treatment to be continued then the situation changes significantly, provided that she still has legal capacity, and that her judgment is not being impaired by clinical depression. Ending treatment could simply be a matter of acceding to a patient's autonomous desire, and allowing the natural trajectory of a disease to take its course. In such a case there could be an added implication to the effect that continued treatment would constitute an act of battery.[23]

It is not clear that any moral distinction can be drawn between acts of withholding or withdrawing treatment, as both types of activity can fall within the scope of normal clinical activity. Legally, especially in the US, it is sometimes more difficult to stop treatment once it has been started than to decide not to begin a treatment at all, but the same does not necessarily apply in the UK. Each case has to be assessed according to the particular circumstances. Nonetheless, in determining an appropriate course of action, clinical decisions ought to be made in cognisance of relevant legal, moral and medical considerations.

The distinction between right and wrong is not always easy to determine, and while practice guidelines can be referred to so as to help determine which course of action ought to be followed, this method is certainly not infallible and scope remains for making clinical judgment based on the presenting facts of a case. While guidelines are likely to be drawn up by reference to what is legal, as well as what might or might not be clinically appropriate, an understanding

of legal and ethical issues on the part of the practising clinician is clearly worth
having, especially in areas of clinical activity where there is an known or imminent risk of death. Accountability in terms of clinical intervention is sometimes
judged according to whether a patient lives or dies, whereby death is viewed as
a type of failure. But that is not a helpful attitude to take unless, however, there
is reason to question someone else's judgment or ability. In which case 'blowing
the whistle' to report significant failures could be ethically appropriate in
protecting the future needs of patients.

Resuscitation orders, the role of the courts, and the doctrine of double effect

Do not attempt resuscitation orders (DNARs) are sometimes issued by responsible clinicians recognising that presenting signs and symptoms indicate that
attempts at cardiopulmonary resuscitation may either be unsuccessful or cause
unnecessary suffering for the limited prospect of benefit being derived from
efforts to restart the heart. This is a judgment call that only the clinician at the
bedside is able to make. However, complications can easily ensue that bring into
question the rights of the patient, the presence and validity of advance statements, and the role of a spouse or member of an immediate family. DNARs can
be contentious and if, for example, bringing a capacitous patient into the discussion would cause potential harm to the extent that it could outweigh the
benefits of involvement, then it would be quite reasonable to exercise therapeutic privilege.[24]

Best practice would suggest that where close family is present it should be
consulted and reasons given for why a particular decision is being made or why
something is being considered. DNARs are sometimes issued without consulting
a patient, and if the patient does have capacity then this is not an ethically desirable practice. In cases of incapacity, involving the family is likely to be
appropriate but at present it is not a requirement. A valid advance statement on
the other hand is different, and if circumstances pertain in the manner that a
patient had previously described, then such wishes ought to be respected. To
ignore them would be to over-ride patient autonomy, and hence unethical and
potentially unlawful.

Questions often arise about whether and when to refer to the courts, and
some clinicians take this route in order to avoid possible blame for wrongdoing
should things not turn out as planned. This may be advisable, especially in
terms of defensive medicine, and may at times be strictly necessary, but the
courts should not be resorted to inappropriately and they do not normally need
to be involved in routine clinical decisions.[25]

The doctrine of double effect (DDE) is a legal device that has its origins in the
fourteenth century, and therefore it is not an exaggeration to describe it as
medieval. But for better or for worse, the concept is enshrined in English law
and is unlikely to be discarded any time soon. Proving intent plays a major part
in criminal (as opposed to civil or common) law decisions, and the DDE is
intended to weed out cases where there is a deliberate intent to kill from those
where there is an intention merely to do the best for a patient and provide
appropriate treatment even if there is an unintended consequence of hastening

death. When life is shortened as a result of administering treatment (such as opiate analgesics) death is perhaps only brought forward by a matter of days or hours, and this possibility is discussed more fully in Chapter 6 (on sedation). The DDE is a relatively cumbersome device to use, and it is questionable whether or not it always separates wrongful doing from standard clinical practice,[26] although in essence it is meant to differentiate the foreseeable but unintended consequences of an act from a deliberate intent to either kill or maim.[27]

Clinical perspectives

It is time now to consider some of these issues in a more applied setting, i.e. from the point of view of the practising clinician. Clinical decision making at the end of life entails four fundamental requirements.

1 The relevant evidence-based knowledge regarding outcomes for the particular interventions, for example 'what are the chances of surviving a cardio-pulmonary resuscitation (CPR) attempt?'. This may be difficult as often the evidence is lacking or weak, or not easy to apply to the patient concerned.
2 To be able to recognise the dying phase of life and to take the appropriate action. At this stage efforts are no longer aimed at cure or even prolongation of life. Failure to recognise that this stage has been reached results in unnecessarily burdensome investigations or treatment, and then appropriate steps are not taken to ensure a comfortable and supported death (Ellershaw and Ward, 2003).
3 Appropriate communication skills encompassing the ability to actively listen, explore ideas, concerns and expectations, and sensitively explain the reasons for coming to decisions. It often seems that coming to the correct moral or clinical decision is relatively straightforward, but communicating this and reaching agreement with all those involved (both professional and non-professional) results in dispute and breakdown in care.
4 Ensuring effective processes are in place (including members of a multidisciplinary team) to reach agreement over complex, moral decisions.

The 'art' for healthcare professionals is to develop the trusting relationship with patients and those close to them, to gain understanding of the issues faced, and to work together in weighing the benefits and burdens of an intervention against the need to respect patient autonomy.

The role and limitations of autonomy have been discussed earlier in this chapter, and it is clear that professionals have a duty to honour competently made advance statements. However, knowing of the existence of such statements and exploring patients' other wishes in advance is a challenge that professionals need to meet. Studies have shown that formal enquiry can uncover significant amounts of information and also increase patients' confidence in the healthcare team (Murtagh and Thorns, 2003; Sayers et al., 2001).

In terms of assisted dying, research in Canada indicates that 8.5% of hospitalised cancer patients have a serious and pervasive desire for death (Chochinov et al.,

1995). Such a figure is likely to vary according to the phrasing of the question, the clinical condition of the patient, the surroundings, and a host of countless other factors that impact on social, psychological and spiritual well-being. Clinical experience suggests that requests for life to be ended prematurely, in specialist palliative care, do occur regularly, though not too frequently, in practice.

The following are the main reasons for such requests.

- **A cry for help:** Patients may have unresolved concerns in terms of physical symptoms, social, psychological or spiritual issues. This leaves them feeling fearful and unsupported. At a time of great uncertainty patients are left feeling out of control as they have insufficient information or opportunity to express their needs.
- **A feeling that suffering may be prolonged:** Symptoms tend to increase as death becomes closer, especially in advanced cancer. However, patients may have an impression that they are likely to remain in this poorly condition for a lengthy period of time when often the case is that their prognosis at this stage is quite short. Sensitive exploration and correction of misperceptions can improve this element of their distress.
- **Depression:** In Chochinov's study there was a strong link between a desire to hasten death and clinical depression. However, the diagnosis of depression is not straightforward as the end of life approaches. Many factors that indicate depression may also be part of the adjustment to situations that patients now find themselves in. Similarly, interventions that work at other times of life may not be appropriate in the last few weeks.
- **A reasoned and logical approach that life no longer has a purpose or sufficient quality:** Having excluded (or treated) the situations described above, we are left with a small number of patients who are quite clear that their needs would be best met by their lives being ended prematurely.

In Chochinov's study, he describes two patients who maintained their serious and pervasive desire for death two weeks later. Interestingly, they were quite different. The first was a 72-year-old man who had troublesome symptoms, with signs of depression, and who was isolated from his wife who was elderly and unable to visit. The second was a 61-year-old lady with no troublesome symptoms and a supportive family. She recognised her life was coming to an end, she hoped to die whilst she still retained her mental competence, reasonable bodily self-control and what she perceived as an acceptable level of dignity.

The responsibilities for the professional when faced with requests to end life are to follow the above list of reasons by using the communication skills of listening and explanation, helping to re-establish the patient in a position of control of their situation by careful assessment of troublesome symptoms and the presence of depression. This will satisfactorily relieve the distress of the majority of patients without recourse to active measures to end life. For the small number that fall into the final category, primary responsibility lies in acknowledging a patient's wishes and continuing to provide the best palliative care available.

Once a patient enters the palliative phase of their illness, a number of investigations and interventions become unnecessary. This may range from simple recording of blood pressures to major procedures such as CPR. The essence of decision making in these situations is accurate recognition of the dying phase. In this phase there may be no reasonable methods available to prolong life or maintain it at a sufficient quality, in considering quality of life estimation, patients' attitudes and ideals need to be considered. As discussed above, respect for the patient's autonomy may conflict with the professional's own autonomous values in not inflicting any unnecessary harm.

Discussions need to centre around the general situation in which patients find themselves rather than focusing on a specific issue being discussed. For example, if CPR is felt to be futile owing to the generally frail state of the patient, a better starting point for discussion would be the patient's condition, and what would need to be done in terms of ensuring comfort, the appropriate place of care, and support for family and for those close to the patient, and so on. Having assessed patient (and family) understanding of these issues, it then becomes easier to move on to interventions that are no longer appropriate, such as CPR. In fact, often by this stage the situation is so clear to all involved that the CPR question becomes self-evident.

There is often a concern from professionals that the 'final injection' or last dose increase of opioid or sedative caused the death of a patient. There is also a popular perception that this is routine practice at the end of life (Corner, 1997). As far as can be gathered from evidence from clinical experience in palliative care, the DDE would appear to be more of a theoretical than a practical concern. It is a difficult area to investigate convincingly. However, the evidence as it stands suggests that the DDE is rarely required, even in specialist palliative care practice (Sykes and Thorns, 2003a). As death approaches it is likely that symptoms will worsen, and so to maintain comfort, doses of medication may need to be increased. But having to double doses of opioids in the last week of life is unusual in specialist palliative care, so if professionals find themselves having to invoke the DDE or make significant increases in opioid or sedative doses then this is a clear indication for seeking specialist advice (Thorns and Sykes, 2000). Nonetheless, professionals should feel supported that the law recognises the need to provide a patient with comfort at the end of life, even if there is a risk that life may be shortened,[28] despite all the media attention on some high-profile cases (Horton, 2001).

Notes to Chapter 4

[1] At the time of writing a case is going to appeal based on a competent patient's right to demand continued treatment for a terminal condition, even though the medical prognosis is extremely poor. The case centres on a patient's desire to continue to receive artificial feeding and hydration, and to be protected from the actions of clinicians who might consider it inappropriate to continue this treatment in the final stages of a progressive terminal disease. This case may have future implications as regards medical futility and the continuation of treatment, including artificial feeding and hydration. Cf. Dyer (2004).

[2] This does not presuppose that clinicians are poor at making judgments on behalf of their patients – often they are especially well placed to be able to offer advice to a family, and to make decisions for critically ill patients in their care. But being in this position does not confer absolute rights or powers to make decisions irrespective of the wishes of others. Professional autonomy has its limits and must be seen to show

respect for the rights of others, including the personhood of an unconscious or legally incapacitated patient.

3 In the USA there is something called the *Living Will Registry* – a national computerised database accessible to all medical service providers containing details of advance directives and names of health proxies for everyone registered: www.uslivingwillregistry.com.

4 Cf. The Mental Capacity Bill (2004) issued by the Department for Constitutional Affairs (Part One § 9): www.dca.gov.uk/menincap/legis.htm.

5 *Ibid.* (Part Two §§ 43–57).

6 For example, the Netherlands and Belgium legalised PAS in 2001–2, and Oregon passed a law to this effect in 1997 (see: www.ohd.hr.state.or.us/chs/pas/pas.cfm) (however, this law has since been the subject of a federal legal challenge by the US Attorney General). Also, forms of euthanasia have recently been made legal in France (see Spurgeon (2004)).

7 For example, the term 'non-voluntary' is sometimes used in place of 'involuntary' in those cases where patients lack capacity; both terms could be taken to include cases of withholding or withdrawing treatment.

8 Cf. www.the-shipman-inquiry.org.uk/home for information on the inquiry set up to investigate procedures for reporting death, the workings of coroners' courts, etc.

9 Cf. British Medical Association (2001); British Medical Association (2003: Chapter 11); General Medical Council (2002). At the time of writing, GMC guidelines are subject to judicial review in the High Court. Cf. www.gmc-uk.org.

10 In some states, under the US legal system patients are kept alive for many years in PVS even though there is no hope of them ever making a recovery. The Bland ruling (*Airedale NHS Trust v. Bland 1993 All ER 821*) sought to ensure that the same should not be allowed to happen in England and Wales.

11 The view of the editor and both contributors is such that they do not advocate legalising euthanasia or physician-assisted suicide in the UK. Among other things they maintain that there are other and more important issues that need to be dealt with in terms of care of the elderly and care of the terminally ill (e.g. improving access to specialist provision of pain control, and clarification of the law in relation to the use of sedation). For a survey of arguments against PAS see Keown (2002).

12 For example, *The Death with Dignity Act (Oregon)* (1997) Administrative rules. Cf. www.ohd.hr.state.or.us/chs/pas/pas.cfm.

13 Cf. *The Termination of Life on Request and Assisted Suicide (Review Procedures) Act (Netherlands)* (2001): www.healthlaw.nl/eutha_e.html.

14 Study of this topic falls under the heading of 'thanatology', about which there is a reasonable quantity of literature (cf. Morgan (1997). The person credited with initiating wider study of this subject is Elisabeth Kübler-Ross, who died herself, after a long period of illness, in August 2004.

15 Cf. www.nejm.org.

16 Some well-known cases, such as that of Mrs Diane Pretty, brought the subject to the fore in terms of public debate. For an insight into some of the complexities of this case see the House of Lords ruling (2001): www.parliament.the-stationery-office.co.uk/pa/ld200102/ldjudgmt/jd011129/pretty-1.htm.

17 *See* Chapter 2.

18 For example, Queens Bench Division: adjudication re Mrs Diane Pretty § 37 [2001] EWHC Admin 788.

19 For a review of legal reasoning in analytic jurisprudence see Coleman and Shapiro (2004: Chapters 3–4).

20 See Shapiro (2002) for a fuller discussion on the relationship between law and society and how legal positivism is the only legal theory that may be said to have general acceptability.

21 On the other hand, 'watchful waiting' to see how a disease progresses or doing nothing because to attempt to do anything further would be futile, is not the same thing.

22 Cf. Re B (adult refusal of medical treatment) *Ms B v. an NHS Hospital Trust* [2002] EWHC *429; see also (2002) Medical Law Review. 10:* 201–26.

23 That is, refrain from involving a competent patient in a decision not to resuscitate on the grounds that to do so would not be in a patient's best interests, perhaps because of being in a condition of extreme physical or psychological frailty.

24 This topic is best approached by reviewing case studies, and so further discussion is deferred until Part Two.

25 One of the best known cases that hinges on an interpretation of the DDE is that of *R. v Cox* [12 BMLR 38, 1992].

26 That is, the DDE applies where the action is good or at least morally neutral independent of its consequences. The intention of the agent is thus solely to produce the good effect; the bad effect can be foreseen, tolerated and permitted but not intended by the agent.

27 *R vs Adams* (1957) Crim LR 365.

Chapter 5

Questions of autonomy and rights

Domains and definitions

Essentially, autonomy is a state of being self-governing, such as when someone is able to exercise free will and liberty in making a personal (medical) decision. Medical autonomy is considered to be a right – the right to determine what does (or does not) happen to one's body. However, autonomy is not necessarily an absolute right and in the context of patient rights it is worth considering what limits exist as to its scope. To do this it will be necessary to examine what it means to have a right (to anything), what implications flow from being in possession of that right and what a right 'is', which in itself is not immediately obvious.

In order to claim enjoyment of a right one must first be eligible, and criteria for eligibility vary. Eligibility can be derived simply from being a human being, citizen or person, or can be more narrowly defined by being restricted to membership of a particular group or profession. Doctors and lawyers, for example, have rights or privileges not normally enjoyed by the general public; patients too have rights, which may be different from those of a doctor or lawyer. However, categories of eligibility can overlap, and it is possible for someone to belong to more than one group or classification and simultaneously to have the corresponding rights (e.g. as a human being, a citizen, a patient, and so forth). But the question of eligibility is not the only complicating factor.

To argue that by virtue of being human one ought not to be denied a certain right is to argue in support of something being a basic human right. But if an entitlement claim is with respect to something specific, such as healthcare service provision, it involves making a different kind of claim. To uphold that claim one first has to establish that the entitlement is a right, and second, in order for it to be meaningful, to ensure that the means are available to secure enjoyment of that right. In recognition of factual differences within or between countries, rights to healthcare service provision can be context driven and are not necessarily universal. Generalisable claims, such as a global right to healthcare, are notoriously difficult to sustain.

Medical care in the UK is enjoyed free at the point of delivery, and there are few grounds of eligibility that have to be satisfied.[1] Most but not all healthcare services are therefore available by right to citizens in the UK under the auspices of the National Health Service (NHS).[2] But by way of contrast, the situation is entirely different in the United States, where grounds for eligibility are mainly socio-economic. This is because patient rights are constrained by limits in access to health insurance, and limiting criteria laid down by government, for example, or by a managed care organisation. It is unsustainable and factually incorrect to claim as universal something that cannot be enjoyed by most if not all persons, and so as far as healthcare is concerned in the USA, the right to healthcare is very much conditional and hence not universal. Preconditions limit the right to such an extent that access to healthcare becomes difficult to defend as a right, other than as a point of moral principle or something to which society may want to aspire.

In general, a right to healthcare is relative to levels of distribution that can deliver the appropriate goods and services, and political will is also needed in order to ensure their delivery. Almost all governments find it hard to meet the demand for healthcare services, whatever the prevailing local or regional politics. However, to claim that a right such as healthcare has been denied either to oneself or to others may be relatively easy if the NHS, for example, were to deny a treatment that was subject to statutory provision. But more often, to prove why something is a right in the first place and determining how best a claim can be upheld can be much more difficult.

The right to healthcare is an example of a positive right, but negative rights, such as the right to be free from coercion or undue interference, can also be claimed as rights. Rights such as the right to marry and found a family and the right to life are now embedded within the Human Rights Act 1998, and in the UK this is the Act that since implementation in 2000 has broadly defined the parameter of legal rights. While not all rights can be categorised as either positive or negative, the positive–negative distinction is an oft-used method of contrasting various categories of rights and although its value is limited, the classification should not be ignored.[3]

The moral versus legal distinction may have greater significance and while a right may be ethically desirable, it may not be legally enforceable. Conversely, if a right is upheld in law, it may be presumed though not proven that it is also morally sustainable. The language of rights makes this type of distinction and declarations, for example, usually concern moral principle and are thus broadly framed. Conventions are often more detailed and akin to legal agreements, hence open to challenge in court (such as in the European Court of Human Rights in Strasbourg) were, for example, a government to fail to adhere to the terms of an article or code.[4] In sum, it is incoherent simply to argue that 'a right is a right is a right', or that all rights are necessarily universal. Most rights are conditional, not absolute, and without diluting their moral status, it makes sense to recognise that there are unavoidable boundaries and limitations to rights holding and entitlement. Also, it is both reasonable and pragmatic to accept the possibility that rights can clash with one another, which matter will be discussed shortly.

Rights at the end of life

The Human Rights Act 1998 is the UK enactment of a European bill of rights, the influence of which is far-reaching. The Act does not define what a right is in and of itself, but by specifying the spheres of activity that fall within its compass it broadly determines how rights impact on institutions and on the lives of individual citizens. While the Act does not define parameters for the provision of medical care, some articles are applicable and they provide a logical background against which to position an assessment of rights at the end of life. While legal statute is not the vehicle for defining all there is to say about a right, the Act provides a starting point for assessing how rights impact both on vulnerable patients and on the practising professional.

Relevant provisions from Schedule One of the Human Rights Act 1998 include the following.

- **Article 1** refers to the 'dignity of the human person [which] must be respected and protected'.
- **Article 2** states that the 'right to life shall be protected by law'.
- **Article 5** states that 'no-one [shall be] deprived of liberty save in [certain] cases [e.g.] lawful detention (of) ... persons of unsound mind'.
- **Article 8** upholds the 'right to respect for private and family life'.
- **Article 14** prohibits 'discrimination on grounds of sex, race, colour, language, religion, political or other opinions, national or social origin, association with a national minority, property, birth or other status'.[5]

Article 1 is fundamental in that everything else flows from being in possession of it and having it respected by others (e.g. by those in a position of responsibility towards a terminally ill patient). It encompasses all other domains, it is generic in nature, and it does not have a specific field of application. However, it is worth discussing the use of the word 'dignity'. Dignity is a somewhat abstract notion and can have different meanings and interpretations, particularly as applied to death and dying. Death with dignity for one person can mean being allowed to choose the time and manner of one's death. However, it could just as well be argued by another person that 'such matters do not lie within human hands and should not be subject to individual choice'. Furthermore, dignity in death could mean allowing nature to take its course with a minimum amount of invasive medical intervention, and/or being allowed to observe the basic tenets of one's religion.

It would be wrong to oversimplify this discussion, but if dignity in life means showing respect for the needs and aspirations of others, then dignity in death is a logical extension of that concept. Therefore if dignity in life has meaning, by inference, it also has meaning in relation to death,[6] in that it makes little sense to talk about dignity as referring to something different during life from what it means in relation to death. In Eastern religions such as Buddhism, life is regarded as a form of preparation for death, and in effect, death need not be considered to be a right at all but rather can be seen as the final event in life. Thanatology (the study of death and dying) should not be exclusively biased towards a Western viewpoint, and it is helpful to consider other viewpoints to help gain a more complete understanding. Social policy ought similarly to reflect the multicultural nature of the population it encompasses, and it is unethical to disempower any person simply by reason of adherence to a particular pattern of belief. In short, demonstrating respect for human dignity is synonymous with demonstrating respect for persons, and to argue otherwise is to challenge the whole basis of respect for autonomy and rights.

Article 2 deals with the right to life, although from the full wording of this article it is clear that its primary domain is criminal law, not medical decision making.[7] The courts declined to accept that a right to die can be upheld under this Article and it so does not fall within the scope of the provisions of the Act.

In the case of a terminally ill patient it usually falls to the medical professional to make decisions that impact upon the manner and time of death, and such decisions basically rest on the shoulders of one individual. As noted in Chapter 3, where possible, decision making should be a team process in consultation with the family (and of course, if competent, the patient). Such discussion should take place before a decision to terminate active treatment is taken, whether or not the only likely clinical outcome is death. There is little evidence to support rights claims pertaining specifically to death, and while such a notion does not diminish the concept of respect for the dead in any way, it is more logically and ethically coherent to talk about rights as pertaining to the living.

Nevertheless, what happens in the days and months leading up to death is crucial, and quality of life not quantity of life is often the main issue. It is because of this that active treatment might not always be in a patient's best interests.[8] While decision making is influenced by matters of clinical judgment, the switch from active treatment to palliation only has legal and ethical implications, and no one's rights should be infringed by the act of switching. Denying treatment that a patient wants and needs is both legally and ethically problematic, but it is inappropriate and unethical to administer unwanted treatment with no prospect of a beneficial outcome.

The right to life is an essential part of decisions made near the time of death, and while respecting autonomous patient rights, it is still the primary duty of doctors to take reasonable steps to try to preserve the life of a patient. Patient rights at or near the time of death are crucially important to defend, and denial of the basic right to self-determination in its most egregious form amounts to wilful killing.[9] Upholding the right to life does not have to fly in the face of reason by trying to take heroic measures and avoid the inevitable, but if the right is denied, then serious consequences should be expected to follow.

Article 5 has implications for patients with mental rather than physical illnesses, and the Article does not directly relate to the subject at hand, except perhaps in cases where a dangerously violent mental health patient is suffering from a terminal medical condition.

Article 8 pertains to all citizens, and having respect for this provision should prevent state powers from being unreasonably and unlawfully exercised. This includes but is not limited to decisions made around the time of death, and under the Act scope is allowed for the provision to be invoked 'for the protection of health and morals, or for the protection of the rights and freedoms of others'.[10]

Article 14 is of major importance in relation to the demonstration of respect for patient values, to decisions made on behalf of someone who is incapacitated, and to the whole way in which care is administered. To discriminate unfairly and to show lack of respect for the values and beliefs of patients is unethical and unprofessional and patients needing palliative care treatment can be from either sex, of any age, and belonging to any religion, race or ethnic group. The provision of medical care may never be entirely free of bias, and wholly non-discriminatory attitudes and conduct may be an unattainable ideal. However, *not* to strive towards such a goal is perhaps as unethical as actively to harbour prejudice and unfair discriminatory attitudes. To aspire toward a non-discriminatory ideal, and to do that which is within one's power to protect patients from harm caused by wrongful discrimination is an important part of good clinical practice. Furthermore, over time, respecting patients' values may be capable of incrementally raising standards of care.

Autonomy, rights and the patient–doctor relationship

The basis of the relationship that exists between doctor and patient has changed greatly within a relatively short period of time. A mere generation ago patients probably had lower expectations in terms of 'cure', medical paternalism was more or less 'the norm' and the authority of the medical 'expert' was rarely called into question. Similarly, patient rights was an unfamiliar concept, autonomy was little discussed and – rightly or wrongly – the medical profession enjoyed high social status. There was little sense of partnership or shared responsibility in the provision of healthcare, and patients and medical students alike tended to live in fear of a senior clinician. Raised awareness of patient autonomy and rights is at the root of many of these changes; it forms part of a wider pattern of social change and provides the background to the discussion that follows.

One should not assume too much in terms of attitudes and behaviour, either from patients or clinicians; in the modern healthcare environment patients can sometimes be demanding and aggressive, and physicians too can be unhappy, especially if overly constrained by protocols, bureaucracy and scarce resources. Essentially, the philosophical dimensions of the patient–physician relationship have to do with limits of autonomy, the basis of shared decision making, and arguments about respective rights, and it is time now to consider how this dynamic directly or indirectly affects care at the end of life. Changes in the relationship have to do with changed roles as well as with changes in perception. The role of the clinician is to act as medical expert, skilled technician, and to some extent as patient advocate under the premiss of a duty of care. However, advocacy does not authorise clinicians to assume knowledge of the wishes of patients that they do not actually possess.

Ethically speaking, a clinician should make an effort to try and ascertain the wishes of a particular patient in relation to a proposed course of action (or inaction), i.e. should not simply act as if 'doctor knows best'. The right to autonomy necessitates some form of reciprocal behaviour, both at macro (social policy) level, and at micro (individual doctor and patient) level. However, the extent to which attitudes of patients affect the care that they receive, and the extent to which being a rights-holder brings measurable benefit are valid topics for investigation and nothing can simply be assumed.[11]

There is little value to be had from being in possession of a right if it makes no physical, emotional or psychological difference to the rights-bearer. For rights to be meaningful they need to benefit society as a whole, and/or the individual holder, and in order for benefits to be derived, some person or body needs to be beholden to provide the means of satisfaction or enjoyment of that right. In the context of terminal illness it may seem illogical to talk about 'enjoyment' of rights, but the failure to show proper respect towards a dying patient has the potential to increase suffering, and cause serious harm to both patients and their families.

The nature of the relationship between carer and cared for, and between clinician and patient is a fundamental component part of the discussion about autonomy and rights.[12] If attitudes are confrontational and adversarial, as can be the case when there is no meaningful or satisfactory relationship, harm can ensue, and there is clearly a line to be drawn between demanding something as one's right and engaging with a person or agency, upon whose services one is dependent, in a meaningful way in order to obtain necessary care.

To overplay the claim towards enjoyment of rights becomes counterproductive if, in the process of pressing a claim, the trust that forms the basis of the relationship is thereby irrevocably damaged. Without trust the relationship is unable to function and the patient remains at the mercy of the clinician or service provider, making it more difficult for doctors to secure the active participation of patients in their care. For rights to be meaningful they have to be respected and/or legally enforceable; but to rely on the force of law and the adversarial system that it embodies is to ignore a key tenet of good medical practice, namely *trust*. Statutory rights need universal respect, but demand for legal protection of a right needs to be enforced with some discretion if the court system is not to be overburdened, and if the doctor–patient relationship is to be allowed to retain even a small element of trust.

The tendency to be dependent upon claiming rights in order to secure a service is set to fail unless the parties involved first try to demonstrate a measure of mutual respect and trust. Rights do not exist in a 'moral-free zone', especially in the medical setting, and basic standards of morality should be expected from key stakeholders, patients and providers alike. As Parekh said in an Oxford Amnesty Lecture (Parekh, 2004), 'Society that relies on rights to ensure moral order is too impoverished to nurture valuable forms of human excellence'. This Aristotelian reference to human excellence is well made, and Parekh's comment does not belittle rights – it serves instead as a reminder that to live in a society dominated by a powerful need to uphold claims to the protection of legal entitlements may not always be an attractive proposition if standards of individual and collective morality thereby come to be ignored.[13] The next task is see if, how and when rights conflict one with another.

Conflicting rights and different types of autonomy

Rights do not provide a panacea for all social ills, but they open up a valuable opportunity in which to engage in both moral and legal discourse. In addition, they create an opportunity for socio-legal analysis by looking at ways in which rights are ordered within society, and prioritised one against another. A society, for example, that ignores the rights of the poor or the disabled and the rights of women or ethnic minorities may be a society that cares little for social justice. But a society that is socially aware may have more equitable distribution of goods and services, and pay greater attention to the needs of those who, for various reasons, are socially disadvantaged. Although it is not important to discuss here the intricacies of political and social agendas towards different types of rights, what is important is to examine how different categories of autonomy interact with different types of rights. This has implications both for the care of the elderly and for the care of the terminally ill, and some examples now follow of how different categories of rights can at times be in conflict one with one another (progressing from the individual to the collective).

Patient autonomy versus clinician autonomy

The right to freedom of thought and expression and the right to be free from undue interference are mutually incompatible if one person holds a strong view as to what is the best course of action to take and seeks to impose that point of view on to another. For instance, a patient's autonomous rights can potentially be over-ridden by a clinician, and there is no reason why a patient should not also hold strong views about right and wrong, and about individual preferences and what happens to her body. If these views do not coincide, autonomy is the concept that gives moral authority to the views of a patient, and however clinically validated clinicians' viewpoints might be, ultimately it is not they who are being treated or their health and well-being that are at issue.

Paternalism (i.e. when clinicians explicitly over-ride the autonomous rights of patients in their care) no longer falls into the category of 'good medical practice'. Therefore, in terms of treatment decisions, the concept of autonomy gives ethical validity to the patient's point of view in the event of disagreement, in spite of an imbalance in terms of knowledge and power; it is difficult for vulnerable patients to protect themselves against a so-called 'authority' figure (assuming, that is, that patients have the necessary capacity with which to uphold their autonomous rights and are able to exercise those rights as an individual).

Inclination is also needed because it is of little use empowering a patient if that self-same person says 'Ok, doc, you know what's best, just do what you have to'. While this can sometimes be a legitimate response for a patient to make, such a response has the effect of re-empowering the clinician and so it has to be an entirely voluntary response from the patient, i.e. void of any sense of coercion.[14] No rights are violated if such a decision is freely and independently made and if a patient is fully aware of the implications of delegating power back to the clinician. However, such re-empowerment should be the exception not the general rule, otherwise the whole process of seeking and obtaining consent to medical interventions loses meaning. Clinicians have autonomy on two separate counts – one, by reason of their qualifications and earned professional status, and two, on account of their own individual rights, freedoms and personhood – and the question is how these rights relate to the autonomous rights of patients. In the event of a healthy patient–doctor relationship few problems are likely to arise, but the dynamic of the patient–doctor relationship can vary considerably and where it breaks down, it is possible for faults to lie on either or both sides. Patients can be unreasonable, demanding and even wholly unco-operative, and clinicians do not lack opportunity to display unpleasant or inappropriate personal or professional traits. No textbook or court of law can change this situation, but what is open to change is the manner in which individuals conduct themselves, and how one individual responds to inappropriate behaviour on the part of another.

To illustrate how patient and professional autonomy can be at odds, some cases that have recently been investigated by the Health Service Ombudsman for England and Wales will next be discussed. They relate to harm caused by failures in communication and informed consent procedure. The role of the Health Service Ombudsman is important in relation to the protection of patient rights, and a formal recommendation made by her office can lead to direct representation to Parliament, with the specific intention of ensuring that harms are not repeated.[15] The office functions as a measure of last resort when all other options have failed; it is not a substitute for taking a case to a court of law, and neither does it function as a court itself. Rather, it provides a way of registering a complaint (which may or may not be upheld), and having it impartially reviewed. If a complaint is upheld then an explanation or apology about what went wrong is likely to be forthcoming, and because of public accountability, there is an expectation that this will indeed happen. If a finding is established in favour of a responsible clinician, then effectively that person's *professional* autonomy has been upheld; if not, then it could be that *patient* autonomy is that which is in need of reinforcement.[16]

A woman was admitted to hospital with abdominal pain and jaundice, and she was given a number of tests which proved inconclusive. The patient was sent home, later to be readmitted with a serious infection from which she subsequently died. Neither the patient nor her husband was aware of the seriousness of the situation or of the fact that the patient may have had an underlying condition that potentially *could* shorten her life (i.e. a malignancy). The patient interview was inadequately performed and nobody checked to see that information (which apparently had been relayed) had been properly understood. The clinical facts, such as were known, were not communicated in a way that a lay person could comprehend; the information 'exchange' was inadequately recorded in the notes, and no steps were taken to ensure that either the patient or the patient's spouse appreciated the possibility of imminent death. A formal complaint was made and partially upheld, and the hospital trust in question eventually gave a written apology to the late patient's spouse.

Had matters been better managed, the clinical situation might have been no different but proper communication and recording of information (such that might have enabled the situation to be addressed sooner) would have been ethically appropriate. It could also have prevented the anger felt by the patient's spouse over how the case was managed overall. In essence, the consultant failed to demonstrate due respect for patient autonomy, and issues of *professional* autonomy (to do what was clinically expedient) trumped the need for good communication and a decision-making process that fully involved the parties most affected.

Clinical uncertainty is an important factor in this case, which can be difficult to handle for patients, as well as for the family (and even for the clinical team). However, not to acknowledge the possibility that presenting signs and symptoms were indicative of a serious malignancy was an error in this case, and the possibility of there being a malignancy should have been communicated to the patient, preferably in her husband's presence. This case shows how patient-centred autonomy was hardly considered by a medical team that appeared to be more concerned about doing a job and thus protecting professional autonomy. Some clinicians argue that raising a matter of considerable uncertainty causes unnecessary harm to a patient, and that such a possibility outweighs potential benefits that might accrue from greater openness and transparency. But that judgment is not theirs to make unless there is sufficient cause for them to exercise their therapeutic privilege.[17]

A second case involves a woman with a history of vascular and heart disease. She underwent vascular bypass surgery on the advice of her cardiologist; she developed post-surgical complications and was subsequently admitted to intensive care. She had further surgery and later died. The patient's daughter was not seeking to prove negligence, but instead was complaining about the informed consent procedure. Her complaint was eventually upheld because the cardiologist had not conveyed sufficient information to the patient about the risks of not having surgery or about the risks of having surgery in this particular case (i.e. in the light of the mother's past medical history). This failure invalidated the consent process, and the senior surgeon made matters worse by failing to offer a satisfactory explanation as to why the patient died post-operatively.

At the time of making the decision to have surgery the patient was fully competent and, as in the previous case, the main issue was the failure to recognise her autonomous rights. This failure concerned her right to be properly informed, as well as the rights of the daughter to have a reasonable explanation about what happened and about why her mother died when she did.

There was no direct criticism of any clinical judgments made, but because the information exchange did not take place properly, harm was done to the extent that the patient herself was unaware of the precariousness of her medical condition. Although lack of information cannot necessarily be proven to be an actual harm, in this instance the daughter was kept in the dark, and as a result suffered additional and avoidable stress following the death of her mother. Patient autonomy lost out to professional autonomy and the desire to respond to clinical considerations, while failing to recognise the rights of interested parties who should have been allowed to play a bigger role in the decision-making process. Finally, maintaining silence after an unsuccessful medical outcome was not a good way to proceed. Greater openness and transparency would almost certainly have limited the harm done by other failures.

Silence at a critical time when explanation is needed may be psychologically damaging, and it can easily lead to legal action being taken against the clinician concerned. Silence leaves in its wake a general feeling of dissatisfaction, even if in clinical terms the final outcome is no different.[18] As Rowe says, speaking from direct personal experience:

> It is not that people sue without medical cause, but that they sue, in part, because they have no place else to go for recognition (from those who should be among the first to give it) that their loved one's life and their loss matter. ... Both doctors and family members might benefit from words and actions that bridge the silence that death leaves behind.
>
> (Rowe, 2002b)

While clinicians may need a certain detachment in order to be able to do their job effectively, that does not absolve them from all responsibility to discuss adverse outcomes, including death, when reasonably requested to do so. To communicate effectively is ethically desirable and it shows respect for autonomy and the rights of persons directly or indirectly under the care of a clinician; it has the potential to minimise harm and the risk of legal action, and overall should be regarded as part of good clinical practice.[19]

Individual rights versus community rights

Localised decisions about allocation of resources are often made from within the context of broader policy decisions. Such decisions are likely to have a political component, and although politics is not the issue here, addressing the question of individual versus community rights is. This means talking about social choices, such as the right to choose the time, manner and place of treatment for individuals versus community rights and the provision of a minimum standard of healthcare services being made available to all. To try and prioritise both only leads to a contradiction and the possibility that neither goal is achieved.

This topic is part of a wider discussion in relation to the type of society in which people want to live. But whether or not it is healthcare that is being discussed, in policy terms, one cannot be pointing in opposite directions at the same time. If consumerism and patient choice are regarded as paramount, then basic concepts of universal access and service provision free at the point of delivery can be put at risk.[20] In the same way, decisions to uphold public interest and the rights of the community at large can jeopardise quality of service provision and people's freedom to choose. These two trends are pulling in opposite directions. Absolute equality of healthcare service provision may be an ideal to which people want to aspire, but it may not be achievable. Historically, the NHS has generally favoured community rights and principles of utility over the rights of individuals, which sometimes resulted in compromise measures over quality of services and the amount of choice patients could reasonably expect.

Policy implications

In terms of policy evaluation and community versus individual rights, the provision of palliative care treatment services has been subject to re-evaluation in England and Wales, and in 2004 the National Institute for Clinical Excellence (NICE) issued guidance detailing what the NHS ought to be doing in providing for this type of care.[21] The policy implications of this can usefully be assessed from the point of view of rights, and in *Improving Supportive and Palliative Care for Adults with Cancer*, the Executive Summary states that:

> In England and Wales cancer accounts for one quarter of all deaths. A diagnosis of cancer and its subsequent treatment can have a devastating impact on the quality of a person's life, as well as on the lives of families and other carers. . . . This Guidance defines service models likely to ensure that patients with cancer, with their families and carers, receive support and care to help them cope with cancer and its treatment at all stages.[22]

The summary document contains a total of 20 key recommendations for improvements, and the current service model relies on cancer networks of partnership organisations, combining both the voluntary and statutory sectors. Networks are meant to work in partnership with provider organisations and multidisciplinary teams, but at present cancer service provision is fragmented and the needs of patients and patients' carers are generally subsumed under a greater need to provide more general types of care. The new system, when it is implemented, will have more of an individualistic approach,[23] and it will be interesting to see how this fits with the older, more community-focused approach towards the provision of specialist services.

The guidance expresses the need for better face-to-face communication, access to better quality of information for patients, the provision of psychological and social support services, rehabilitation services, complementary therapy services, and for more comprehensive palliative care service provision overall. Mechanisms for the provision of palliative care alone (to say nothing of other types of service) are not yet in place, and as the guidance acknowledges, 'Many of the recommendations . . . are critically dependent on workforce development – the appointment of additional staff and the enhancement of knowledge and skills of existing staff'.[24] Policy implementation may take time to bring into effect and policy contradictions of the type indicated will need to be resolved.

The recommendations offered are nonetheless valuable, and go a long way towards trying to meet deficiencies in the current system of service provision. However, while society as a whole will benefit from having better care facilities available when and where they are needed, it still cannot be said that such services can be enjoyed as a legal right. There will be a raft of changes needed in order to be able to see this kind of strategy through to fulfilment. These changes are rights based, and the overall effect is that personal autonomy is likely to be reinforced. This is to be welcomed, but expressions of social choice always imply some kind of trade-off, and this contemporary example of a rights shift is surely no exception.

By definition, healthcare is delivered one patient at a time, and policy decisions taken at macro level eventually filter down to individual episodes of care, such as when a patient is admitted for hospice care in the later stages of terminal illness. In terms of autonomy and rights and the treatment of terminal illness, perverse factors sometimes come into play that impact, for example, on the professional autonomy of a prescribing physician as well as on the rights of an individual patient (to receive care at a critical time of life).

To illustrate this point, an example that came to public attention in 2001–2 is described here concerning the availability of a drug called Herceptin (trastuzumab). Herceptin is a licensed drug with 'proven' efficacy in treating aggressive forms of breast cancer in post-menopausal women, in certain cases extending life by a matter of years. As with many new-generation drugs, it is considerably more expensive than the older generation drug that it supersedes. However, it is not just a replacement for an old drug such as tamoxifen, and neither is the issue just one of comparing a brand-named drug against a new generic equivalent. Herceptin came under scrutiny by NICE when the Institute was charged with trying to tackle disparities that existed in terms of the drug's availability. NICE was seeking to help establish a national policy and give clear guidance as to when the drug could be prescribed (i.e. within the NHS); to do this it needed to carry out scientific analysis of *clinical* effectiveness, and perform an economic analysis on potential *cost*-effectiveness as that is the main function of the organisation.[25] However, a particular problem arose in during the 18 months that NICE took to perform its evaluation, patients were being denied access to the drug because pharmacy advisors did not want to authorise payment for an expensive drug with 'uncertain efficacy', and that could later be withdrawn from general use. A centralised decision was being sought for informing local policy decision as to availability for this treatment. Unfortunately, while policy was being formulated some patients would have died for want of treatment by a fully licensed drug (albeit in limited circulation).

Particular inequities occurred as a result of this situation having arisen but in doing ethical analysis on such matters, one also has to consider whether public interest is better served by allowing the availability of drugs to be influenced by local factors, with no clear unequivocal guidance as to use or availability, or whether it is fairer temporarily to deny treatment to one group of patients, so that a larger (later) group of patients can then derive benefit. On this occasion utility prevailed, sanctioning harm for some patients in the interests of promoting a greater good. The drug is now generally available,[26] although during the period of assessment the autonomous rights of the practising professional were restricted, and the rights of individual patients were also curtailed to the extent that for some, life was shortened as an indirect consequence of the evaluation process.

There would be inequity in one group of patients being allowed access to a drug (e.g. in an affluent area), while a larger group of patients (in a poorer area) went without. But as a counter-argument, the common good would not be served well by allowing unrestricted access to a drug that was so costly that overall public provision of healthcare suffered in consequence. In the herceptin case, NICE did not fail in its duty; likewise, the Department of Health discharged its responsibility to the public, and a defined group of cancer patients now has access to a drug that has the potential to extend life by a matter of years.[27]

In summary, if the rights of an individual always trump the rights of the community there can be a general sense of inequity if affluence not clinical need is the criterion for determining whether or not a patient has access to a new treatment. Professional autonomy may be affected but it is not undermined by the formulation of clinical guidance that goes on to become national policy. However, the rights of the community are potentially affected in that a delicate balance has to be formed between the harms and benefits that can be suffered or enjoyed by different groups of people. The clinician is often the only person able to form a judgment about the needs of particular patients, but individual clinicians do not have access to all data that go into the formation of policy, and so it is not irrational for there to be intermediate layers of decision making, such as that performed by NICE. Analysing the rights implications of policy decisions is (or should be) beneficial but at the same time it has to be recognised that it forms just one element in a larger decision-making process. That process is diminished if the ethical dimensions are not addressed at all, and while the herceptin case can be assessed in different ways, it establishes that these types of decisions are indeed complex and cannot necessarily be made at the bedside.

Autonomy and rights provide a method of ethical analysis that can be helpful if not indispensable in determining standards of best practice, and protecting individual, vulnerable patients. These concepts thus provide a useful bench-mark, but they can easily conflict with other agendas and other ethical criteria such as justice (which was the main ethical criterion in the case concerning the availability of herceptin). Autonomy and rights should not be relied upon to provide an absolute gold standard, against which all other measures are assessed. Autonomy and rights have natural (inherent) limitations but are nonetheless valuable concepts that play an increasingly important role in medical decision making, and problems that do arise need to be analysed from a social and ethical and not just a clinical perspective.

Notes to Chapter 5

1 Service provision is generally dependent on being first registered with a local general practitioner, which means first having an address.

2 The right to receive treatment does not extend as far as the right to receive *any* treatment. The government, strategic health authorities, primary care trusts and the individual clinician each have various rights to determine treatments that are available and what treatment should be offered to which patient.

3 Cf. Shue (1996: Chapter 2).

4 Cf. Symonides (2003: Chapter 1).

5 Cf. The Human Rights Act 1998, The Stationery Office, London: www.legislation. hmso.gov.uk/acts/acts1998/19980042.htm. The remaining Articles have no *direct* relevance.

6 Cf. Macklin (2003). The author of this article takes an alternative view about the concept of dignity in death.

7 The Article reads as follows: 'Everyone's right to life shall be protected by law. No one shall be deprived of his life intentionally save in the execution of a sentence of a court following his conviction of a crime for which this penalty is provided by law' [Article 2.1] ; 'Deprivation of a life shall not be regarded as inflicted in contravention of this Article when it results from the use of force which is no more than absolutely necessary a) in defence of any person from unlawful violence; b) in order to effect a lawful arrest or to prevent the escape of a person lawfully detained; c) in action lawfully taken for the purpose of quelling a riot or insurrection' [Article 2.2]. *Ibid*. Note 5.

8 Administering treatment with little prospect of a positive outcome can leave patients prone to unreasonable harm, and thus poorer quality of life. In difficult cases the courts may need to be involved, such as deciding if and when to withdraw artificial feeding and hydration from a patient who has fallen into a permanent vegetative state. Under current English law, if a clinical decision is to be made, normally only the responsible physician is able to make it on behalf of an adult patient who lacks capacity.

9 Decisions surrounding the time and manner of death are going to be affected by the outcome of the Shipman Inquiry and any subsequent changes of procedure.
Cf. Third Report *Death Certification and the Investigation of Deaths by Coroners* (2003) Command Paper CM. 5854: www.the-shipman-inquiry.org.uk/thirdreport.asp.

10 *Ibid*. Note 5 [Article 8.2].

11 A common law review of autonomy and consent is to be found in the next chapter.

12 Cf. BMA (2003: Chapter 1).

13 In Part Two of this book there is the chance to see how moral and clinical dilemmas can be dealt with on a case-by-case basis; the best theories are of little use if they do not perform the job that they are intended to perform.

14 If patients are unaware of the severity of their condition then it is not an appropriate

response for them to be making, indicating a failure to communicate (and hence to comprehend) all the facts.

15 Cf. www.ombudsman.org.uk.

16 The following data has been anonymised; a full version is in the public domain but for pragmatic reasons, the cases here have been summarised.

17 This is when a clinician acts to protect a patient from the harm of being in possession of knowledge that would be likely to cause physical or psychological deterioration in the patient's condition, i.e. to cause a greater harm than *not* having the information. Therapeutic privilege can be used as a justification for paternalism. Used appropriately, it is a check that only the responsible clinician is able to perform.

18 Cf. Rowe (2002a).

19 Bias in relation to power conferred by professional autonomy is not always tilted one way, and case law upholds the autonomous right of patients to make decisions *contrary* to advice offered by their clinicians (cf. *St George's Healthcare NHS Trust v. S* (1998) All ER 673 and *Ms B v. an NHS Hospital Trust* (2002) EWHC 429). The St George's case demonstrates that paternalistic decisions are now indefensible at law.

20 Adverse implications of a system that pays less heed to social justice implications of healthcare provision can be seen in the USA. The American market-driven health economy allows for some sections of the population to have unparalleled levels of care, and for others to suffer significant deprivation. Straight comparisons are difficult because there is no equivalent to the National Health Service in America. The exception is the Veterans Administration health system that is federally run and provides healthcare services for mostly ex-service personnel and their families. Its focus is more utilitarian than the consumerist, individual rights-based healthcare delivery methods applicable to the majority of the American population.

21 Cf. *Improving Supportive and Palliative Care for Adults with Cancer (Executive Summary)*: www.nice.org.uk/Docref.asp?d=110012.

22 *Ibid*. [pp. 3–4].

23 How easy this will be to deliver in a system dominated by quotas and systems of audit and central control that allow little latitude for making allowances for special needs of an individual remains to be seen.

24 *Ibid*. Note 26 [p.13].

25 This is an awkward mix of tasks, but it is how the Institute was first set up and its role is unlikely to change significantly.

26 Cf. National Institute for Clinical Excellence press release (2002) *NICE recommends trastuzumab (Herceptin) for advanced breast cancer* [2002/015]: http://www.nice.org.uk.

27 Any harm done may have been 'incidental' and time-limited, but nonetheless real for those caught in the time-trap of policy formulation, the result of which was a small but unknown number of premature deaths.

Chapter 6

The use of sedation at the end of life

Sedation: the issues and definitions

The need for a peaceful death is generally accepted, incorporating the amelioration of unpleasant symptoms. However, some symptoms can be refractory[1] to clinical efforts at palliation and result in significant distress. Sedation offers one means of dealing with this distress and providing patients and their carers (both professional and informal) with a method of achieving some relief. There are potential risks involved, for example the risk of premature death, that understandably can make professionals reluctant to initiate this type of intervention or run the risk of labelling a symptom as refractory in order to cover up poor skills at palliation.

End-of-life issues often overlap, and such blurred edges make definitions important to ensure that actions and purpose are sufficiently clear to describe the concept concerned. In order to facilitate further discussion and research regarding sedation at the end of life, there is a need for standard definitions and terms to be applied. The current literature is hard to interpret as a result of the variety of definitions employed, and a standard definition of sedation at the end of life is therefore important.

Various phrases have been employed to cover this area of practice, including:

- sedation
- terminal sedation
- sedation for intractable distress in the imminently dying
- end-of-life sedation
- total sedation
- sedation in the final phase
- palliative sedation
- palliative sedation therapy.

Three review articles have considered this area: Chater *et al.* (1998), Morita *et al.* (2002) and Beel *et al.* (2002). In a survey of palliative care physicians, Chater used 'sedation' to mean:

> The intention of deliberately inducing and maintaining deep sleep for the relief of a) one or more intractable symptoms when all other possible interventions have failed, or b) profound anguish that is not amenable to spiritual, psychological, or other interventions, when the patient is perceived to be close to death.

Only 40% of respondents totally agreed with this definition. Chater concluded that 'sedation for intractable distress in the dying' best summed up the concept she was trying to describe.

Beel found that there was no clear definition available and provided a comprehensive list of terms used. The phrase 'terminal sedation', used in 26 of the 63 articles found, was felt to convey a negative message suggesting that sedation was a measure to be used in ending life, which could discourage professionals from using this intervention, when compared with other definitions that capture ideas of managing refractory symptoms. Beel adopted the term 'palliative sedation therapy' that was based on the Chater definition.

Morita (2002) searched the literature and drew out themes that definitions encompassed. He found the following elements to be important:

- the use of sedative medications and/or any intention to reduce patient consciousness
- the aim of achieving symptom palliation
- symptoms should be severe
- the patient's distress should be refractory.

However, he found inconsistencies in terms of degree of sedation, duration and pharmacological properties of medications used, target symptoms and target populations.

It would seem from these discussions that a definition needs to encompass the following:

- an aim to reduce a patient's conscious level with a view to treating a particular symptom or cause of distress
- that the symptom should be refractory to other interventions and intolerable in terms of suffering.

Morita in a personal communication (2004) suggests the following definitions:

1 **palliative sedation therapy**, which is 'the use of sedative medications to relieve intolerable and refractory suffering by a reduction in patient consciousness'
2 **sedation in end-of-life care**, which is 'a therapy that uses specific medications to relieve intolerable suffering from symptoms refractory to other treatment by reducing the level of consciousness of patients receiving end-of-life care'.

For the rest of this chapter I shall use the term 'sedation in end-of-life care'. This will not therefore encompass sedation for temporary procedures.

There is also a need to define components within these definitions such as 'refractory', 'intolerable suffering' and 'end of life'. Chater *et al.* (1998: note 2) define *refractory* as when 'all other treatments have failed'. Quill and Byock (2000) define it as when 'palliative care is available but cannot adequately relieve a patient's suffering'. Cherny and Portenoy (1994) define a situation as refractory if any intervention:

- will not bring adequate relief
- will be associated with intolerable morbidity
- will not bring relief within a reasonable time.

They emphasise the need for expert input into this situation, and these symptoms should be 'refractory' and not simply 'difficult'. Distinctions may need to be drawn between physical symptoms such as pain, which are quite clearly defined, as opposed to more subjective factors such as 'distress' or 'restlessness'.

Defining 'intolerable' is more subjective as this needs to be based on a patient's perception. Only they can determine the effect of a symptom on their quality of life. The healthcare team plays an important role in determining and discussing with the patient the possible interventions and the likely progression of the disease and symptoms. The patient and professional can then weigh up these factors. The resulting individuality of this definition leads to diversity of research findings and likely variances as a result of cultural differences (Fainsinger *et al.*, 2003). Finally, a description should distinguish sedation that is intermittent or temporary against permanent, lighter sedation against deep sedation, and situations where sedation is a side-effect of a specific intervention as opposed to where sedation is the primary intention.

The use of sedation: indications, outcomes and methods

Table 6.1 shows the frequency and length of sedative use.

Table 6.1: Frequency of use of sedation in end-of-life care

Study	Method	Sample size and setting	Frequency of sedation (%)	Length of sedative use (days)	Survival (days)
Ventafridda 1990	Prospective	154 home care	52	2 (median)	Sedated 25 Non-sedated 23 (median)
Fainsinger 1991	Retrospective	100 PCU	16	–	–
McIver 1994	Prospective	20 hospital	25	2.5	–
Morita 1996	Retrospective	143 PCU	48	3.9	–
Turner 1996	Prospective	50 PCU + hospital	88	–	–
Stone 1997	Retrospective	115 PCU + hospital	26	1.3	Sedated 18.6 Non-sedated 19.1 (ns)
Fainsinger 1998	Retrospective	278 PCU	1	1.5	–
Fainsinger 1998	Retrospective	76 PCU	30	2.5	–
Morita 1999	Prospective	157 PCU	45	3	–
Peruselli 1999	Prospective multicentre	401 home + hospital	7–60	–	–
Fainsinger 2000	Prospective multicentre	150 PCU + hospital	4–10	2.6	–

(continues)

Table 6.1: Frequency of use of sedation in end-of-life care *(continued)*

Study	Method	Sample size and setting	Frequency of sedation (%)	Length of Sedative use (days)	Survival (days)
Fainsinger 2000	Prospective multicentre	387 PCU	15–36	1.9–3.2	– –
Chiu 2001	Prospective	251 PCU	28	5 (median)	Sedated 28.5 Non-sedated 24.7 (ns)
Morita 2001	Retrospective	209 PCU	60		Overlapping Kaplan-Meier curves
Sykes	Retrospective	237 PCU	48	–	Sedated 38.6 Non-sedated 14.2 (p<0.001)

Reprinted with permission from Elsevier (*The Lancet* (2003) **4**: 312–18).

It can be seen that the prevalence of sedation varies widely from 1% to 88%. The differences may be explained in part by the definitions of sedation used. In a study including light, temporary sedation or sedation resulting as a side-effect of a more specific treatment, the prevalence is likely to be higher than studies only reporting deep sedation to the point of unconsciousness. In studies reporting a proportionate use of sedation, where the depth of the sedation is titrated according to the desired aim and resulting outcome, the median frequency of use is 45% (Sykes and Thorns, 2003a).[2]

The type and geographical location of the units where studies were performed also appear to influence these figures. Units that have more complex and challenging palliative care clinical problems to face appear to have a higher use of sedation than those that are less specialised. This was the case both in Canada (Fainsinger *et al.*, 2000a), where the specialist palliative care unit had a sedation prevalence of 10% compared with the other units' 4%, and in the UK (Stone *et al.*, 1997), where 31% of hospice patients experienced some degree of sedation as opposed to only 21% of hospital patients. Fainsinger *et al.* (2000b) found that sedation was used more than twice as often in a Spanish palliative care unit than in a comparable Israeli setting, with two South African units coming in between. This finding raises the possibility that the triggers for sedation are culturally determined, although the frequency of sedative use from both centres was within the range seen in palliative care practice. Possible factors that may explain this include attitudes to disclosure, perceptions on what is perceived as a 'good death', and different approaches to balancing the need to maintain the patient's ability to communicate alongside relieving distress.

Indications for sedation

A systematic review found that the syndrome of delirium and agitation in an extremely ill patient was the most common indication for sedative use in cancer palliative care, with a weighted mean of 65%.[3] Breathlessness was the next most frequent reason (weighted mean 26%), and pain next with a weighted mean prevalence of 14%. Table 6.2 shows a more detailed breakdown of these figures.

Table 6.2: Principle types of sedative medication employed and indications for the sedation

Study	Principal types of sedative drugs used		Principal indications for sedation	
Ventafridda 1990	Diazepam	} percentages	Dyspnoea	41%
	Chlorpromazine	} not stated	Pain	39%
	Haloperidol	}	Delirium	14%
			Vomiting	6%
Fainsinger 1991	Not stated		Delirium	63%
			Pain	37%
McIver 1994	Chlorpromazine	100%	Dyspnoea	55%
	(purpose of study)		Restlessness	45%
Morita 1996	Midazolam	55%	Dyspnoea	49%
	Morphine	55%	Pain	39%
	Haloperidol	33%	Malaise	38%
	Diazepam	15%	Agitation	23%
	Scopolamine	13%	Nausea	10%
Turner 1996	Midazolam, clonazepam, lorazepam, diazepam: percentages not stated		Not stated	
Stone 1997	Midazolam	80%		
	Haloperidol	37%		
	Levomepromazine	33%		
	Phenobarbitone	3%		
Fainsinger 1998	Midazolam	100%	Delirium	100%
Fainsinger 1998	Midazolam	91%	Delirium	96%
	Chlorpromazine	9%	Dyspnoea	4%
	Lorazepam	9%		
Morita 1999	Opioids	37%	Delirium/ restlessness	42%
	Midazolam	31%	Dyspnoea	41%
	Haloperidol	31%	Pain	13%
	Diazepam	13%	Vomiting	1%
	Scopolamine	10%	Psychological distress	1%
Peruselli 1999	Not stated		Not stated	

Reprinted with permission from Elsevier (*The Lancet* (2003) **4**: 312–18).

There is a great deal of variation in these figures. This in part must come down to differences in definition, the fact that more than one symptom is usually present at this time of life, as well as differences in skills in managing symptoms. Whilst pain, dyspnoea and vomiting are unequivocal physical symptoms there is some controversy over the place of more existential symptoms such as 'distress', 'anguish' or 'restlessness'. These are hard to define in an objective manner. However, existential or family distress are relatively common reasons for sedation in some countries[4] and may overlap with 'mental anguish'[5] and 'restlessness' (McIver et al., 1994). Alternatively, this may just be what most other studies classify as delirium.

Although identical behaviours may be given different interpretations in different countries, it has been suggested that in respect of existential distress some of the differences may be genuine. This could be a reflection of there being much lower levels of disclosure in information about cancer in some countries than in others. It may also be that a degree of psychological distress appears as the patient's physical deterioration reveals to her a truth which is unmentionable verbally (McIver et al., 1994: notes 12, 8). Such differences make interpretation of the research very difficult and reinforce the need for the existence of universally agreed definitions.[6]

Outcomes from sedation in end-of-life care

The literature indicates that sedative dose is generally titrated against the effect on the patient's distress, just as morphine doses are titrated against a pain response (McIver et al., 1994: note 9). It is rarely the intention to achieve deep sedation to the point of unconsciousness from the start. Sales (2001) describes this approach as 'proportional', where the patient remains conscious whilst achieving an adequate degree of sedation. To effectively titrate the dose of sedative the aims and expected outcomes of the treatment must first be defined. The aim of sedation at this stage of life is to relieve intolerable suffering caused by specific symptoms. The aim is not to end life as this would be euthanasia. The expected outcomes are therefore:

- rapid relief of distress
- the lightest level of sedation possible
- death resulting from the natural course of the disease.

The speed of relief is an important factor as patients have little time left and there may only be one chance to get it right. Furthermore, there are possible though unintentional outcomes that need to be monitored for:

- poor relief of symptoms and hence distress
- over-dosage and risk of complications from this
- sedation that is unnecessarily prolonged or at a level that is too deep
- risk of dehydration or lack of nutrition.

Regular assessment and careful documentation of these factors are therefore required.

It is likely that the greatest fear of health professionals using sedation at the end of life is the risk of causing premature death, and some articles have suggested this may be accepted practice (Billings and Block, 1996). However, a systematic review has disputed this claim (Billings and Block, 1996: note 9). Ten studies that examined length of use of sedation before death found a weighted mean of 2.8 days before death, and this might indicate that sedation resulted in death 2–3 days after commencement or alternatively that sedation is only employed in the last days of life and that death would have occurred at this point regardless. Five studies were also identified that compared survival from admission of sedated and non-sedated patients. None of the studies found a shorter period of survival for the sedated group. This does not prove that sedatives used in this situation have no effect on survival – only a controlled trial could demonstrate this, which would be unethical; the finding could be explained by the fact that patients who go on to require sedation are admitted earlier, hence lengthening their survival from this point. But it does provide reasonable evidence to dispute the claims of slow euthanasia and to counter any fears of precipitating an early death.

Methods of sedation

Sykes (Sykes and Thorns, 2003a: note 9) found the drugs used for sedation in this patient group varied between countries, but midazolam was the most frequently used sedative in eight of the 13 studies that reported on medications and was second most often used in three others. Psychotropic drugs were used frequently, sometimes in conjunction with benzodiazepines, but are the most favoured drug category in only three reports, two using haloperidol and the other chlorpromazine. Opioids were reportedly used as sedatives in two studies. Barbiturates such as phenobarbitone and propofol have been used in resistant cases.

Public and professional perceptions and understanding

A number of studies have examined the views of patients, family and the general public on the use of sedation. The question of differing cultural perspectives was touched on earlier and it is questionable as to how much information from one country can be transferred to another.

Morita *et al.* (2003) studied both Japanese oncologists and palliative care physicians alongside members of the public. In a secondary analysis of two earlier studies it appeared that although physicians differentiated between a deep level of continuous sedation and physician-assisted suicide (PAS)/euthanasia, the public were more likely to link the two. This, it is suggested, indicates that the public is more influenced by outcomes than by intentions. Muller-Busch *et al.* (2003) retrospectively reviewed the notes of patients dying in a German unit. Of the 80 patients (14.6%) receiving sedation at the end of life, there appeared to be a trend for an increasing number of patients to either include a desire for sedation in advance directives or to request sedation themselves, from 18% in 1995 to 34% in 2002. (These numbers are quite small and so the statistical significance must be questioned.)

In a US survey of patients, bereaved relatives and physicians, looking at patient preferences at the end of life, Steinhauser *et al.* (2000) found that decision making (in terms of trust and a physician comfortable in talking about dying, knowledge of what to expect, plus a named proxy decision-maker, and written wishes regarding future treatment) was rated highly by patients. Patients rated being mentally aware much more highly than did healthcare professionals, which the authors suggest demonstrates that physicians may be more willing to sacrifice lucidity for analgesia than patients. Although being pain free was more important than being mentally aware, the difference was only small (93% against 92%).

Chiu *et al.* (2001) found that 90% of families in Taiwan thought sedation to be acceptable, although only just over two thirds were satisfied with the outcome of the sedation. These terms were not defined. Morita *et al.* (1996) asked physicians what their interpretation of patients' and families' wishes were regarding sedation at the end of life. Of the 69 patients, it was felt 4% wanted to be alert even if suffering continued, compared with 2% of families; 50% of patients were thought to want to be alert as far as they could endure suffering, compared with 38% of families. Finally, 46% of patients wanted to be free from suffering even if they became drowsy, compared with 61% of families. This demonstrates the difference between professionals and families in their interpretation over patients' wishes regarding sedation. Tschann *et al.* (2003) demonstrated that the presence of a family member at the time of the death can affect the approach of the healthcare professionals and the treatment offered by increasing the use of comfort care and decreasing the technology. This was a retrospective review of 370 patients dying in a community hospital. A study of Canadian intensive care specialists and coroners highlighted the joint yet conflicting concerns of families that sedation may be a form of physician-assisted death, but also a counter-fear of the risk of further pain or suffering (Hawryluck *et al.*, 2002).

It appears that families are more commonly involved in the decision-making process than patients, yet may have different views from patients. They may be torn between a need to see their relative comfortable and a wish for their relative to avoid drowsiness and perceived shortening of life. This is also supported by qualitative work in Israel looking at relatives' perceptions of terminal restlessness (Bratjman, 2003). Further exploration of public and professional views would be useful in order to set the context for any guidance on information giving and counselling.

The clinical decision-making process

High-profile legal cases involving use of drugs that can potentially shorten life result in a need for healthcare professionals to ensure they can clearly justify both reasoning and process when they employ sedation. The process therefore requires a number of stages to be considered:

- the clinical decision of a situation being refractory, including the exploration of other specialist inputs
- specialist multidisciplinary review
- full information given in a timely and understanding manner

- assessment of capacity and informed consent
- skilled drug use and review, including consideration of the depth and length of sedation
- clear aims and intention of the sedation
- consideration of hydration and nutritional needs
- careful documentation of the above
- introduction of safeguards to prevent abuse.

Some of these points are quite clear. Others, however, need more careful exploration. The question of safeguards will be considered later in the chapter.

Determining refractoriness

The definition of refractoriness was considered earlier in the chapter, together with the need for careful multidisciplinary review. John, the patient in Short case 1 (*see* p.82), had pain that had not been easily managed; whether or not this could be termed refractory is debatable. In a different patient with a better prognosis, more aggressive steps to control the pain would have been appropriate. However, considering John's deteriorating condition and future wishes, such interventions would have placed an unnecessary burden on him. Refractoriness appears to encompass a more subjective, individual influence. This seems reasonable but makes clear criteria or guidelines hard to apply.

Proportionate drug use and review

Achieving a proportionate level of sedation enables the right balance for a patient, providing relief from distress whilst allowing the maximum potential for interaction and awareness of those close to them. Levels of medication therefore require careful titration and may need to be adjusted up or down. For Gill, in Short case 3 (*see* p.82), rapid increases in medication were required to achieve relief from distress – this is rarely required, even in a specialist palliative care unit (Sykes and Thorns, 2003b). The need for sedation also requires regular review, as it may be that in situations like Mary's (*see* Short case 2, p.82) that temporary relief of distress is all that is required. A retrospective study (Sykes and Thorns, 2003b: note 34) showed an increasing pattern of midazolam use over the last week of life from just over 10% of patients six days before death to just over 50% in the last 24 hours. The dose of sedative drug tended to increase during the last week of life. Comparison of doses of sedative and their pattern of use allows practice to be compared between units, and a number of studies have produced such data (e.g. Sykes, 2003b and Stone *et al.*, 1997).

The place of nutrition and hydration

In acute medical situations such as intensive care, any use of sedation is supported by artificial nutrition and hydration. The aim in this situation is to support the patient through the acute phase of the illness through to recovery. In the majority of cases in palliative care the patient is close to death, and so the aim is to maintain comfort and freedom from distress in the last stages of life. However, there are occasions, as discussed earlier, when sedation may be used temporarily to address an immediate problem, and in this situation there may well be a place for artificial hydration in particular.

The arguments around hydration and nutrition in sedation are the same as general issues at the end of life, and the following considerations have to be taken into account:

- the perceptions of patients and families regarding the place of food and water in maintaining life, the social importance of such actions, and the different emphasis placed on these by different cultures
- the differences in the physiological needs of the dying compared to the healthy patient
- consideration of the consequences in terms of benefits and burdens of withholding artificial hydration and nutrition
- whether life will be shortened by withholding such interventions and if so, by how much
- the views of a patient, possibly stated in advance
- a consideration of the approach when artificial nutrition or hydration is already in progress.

Consent

Capacity and the role of relatives

It is a basic moral norm to involve patients in the decision-making process about their future treatments. For this to be effective the patient has to be in possession of the facts regarding that treatment, and to have the ability to process the information and make a reasoned judgment.[7] Specific issues that might impair full patient involvement in decision making regarding sedation at the end of life include:

- impaired cognition affecting understanding and capacity
- the emotionally charged nature of this time of life
- divisions among the healthcare team over ethical concerns
- different perspectives between patients and their families
- misperceptions by patients and families over intentions regarding the use of sedation
- the indication for sedation being likely to interfere with cognition (e.g. delirium, anxiety, depression or intractable symptoms)
- the impairment of decision making the sedation itself will cause.

Guidance from a number of areas calls for the need for informed consent when sedation is used at the end of life.[8] A survey of Canadian palliative care experts showed that 78% involved the patient to some degree in decisions on sedation at the end of life, whilst 96% involved families to some degree. Fifty-seven per cent of respondents found the decision 'somewhat difficult' or 'very difficult' (Quill *et al.*, 1997: note 2). Morita's Japanese study (1999) showed that in all but 4% of 69 patients who received sedation, an explanation was provided either to themselves or their family. The extent of this explanation varied. In 7% both family and the patient were informed of both the possibility of short-ening life and the risk of somnolence; in 48% family members were fully informed but patients were only told of somnolence, and in 41% family members were fully informed but patients were not told of the risk of either somnolence or shortening life.

Examples of phrases used in this study included: 'To relieve your discomfort, you might be a little drowsy' or 'Do you have anything you want to say before you fall asleep?'. The authors also suggested that the atmosphere and non-verbal communication that occurred at the time of decision making helped inform patients of the implications of their decision. Chiu, in a study from Taiwan of 70 patients receiving sedation (Chiu *et al.*, 2001), reported that consent was gained in 43% of cases from both patient and family, and in 50% consent was gained only from the family. The exact content of the informed consent is not documented. It is clear from these studies that practice is not uniform, that there is variation in the process and content of the consent process, and that in some countries families are used as proxies.

Issues to consider when discussing consent

The first step is to ensure that the patient wishes to be involved in decisions around end-of-life issues, and to ascertain their wishes in terms of involving family and friends in information giving and decision making. (The ways of communicating delicate information should be a basic skill in healthcare and will not be expanded on here.) A number of authors (Morita *et al.*, 1999: notes 29, 6; Chan *et al.*, 2004: esp. note 6) have suggested an approach to discussing sedation at the end of life. It is suggested that the following points should be included in any discussion.

- The poor chance of recovery, that death is inevitable, and the severity of present suffering and whether this is physical or existential.
- The need to establish that all palliative methods have been applied before coming to a decision on sedation.
- That the side-effects of sedation may include life-shortening potential and decreased levels of consciousness.[9]
- That the opinion of the multidisciplinary team is that the benefits of sedation should outweigh the burdens.
- That the intention of sedation is to relieve distressing symptoms, and not to cause sedation directly or to shorten life.
- That continuous review be undertaken, and that there is the possibility of discontinuing sedation.

Discussion should also include other end-of-life issues that may be considered appropriate at this time. Cherny and Portenoy (1994: note 7 (p.36)) sum this up with the guidance:

In this situation the clinician should explain that by virtue of the severity of the problems and the limitations of the available techniques the goal of providing the needed relief without the use of drugs that may impair the conscious state is probably not achievable. The offer of sedation as an available therapeutic option is often received as an empathic acknowledgement of the severity of the degree of patient suffering. No patient should have to ask to be killed for persistently unrelieved pain, and contra wise, no patient should be sedated without appropriate consideration of other options and informed consent by the patient or proxy.

The theories and legal position on consent

Alderson and Goodey (1998) reviewed the theories and constructs of consent. The almost routine (and hence meaningless) 'functionalist consent' likened consent to a polite ceremony to enable responsibility to pass from the doctor to the patient. The more factually based 'real consent' requires a defined level of information transfer, thereby allowing standards to be set and assessed. However, neither of these concepts covers the practical situations healthcare professionals are faced with at the end of life. Here, a huge range of complexities are present in a highly charged atmosphere, with patients with poor decision-making and information-retaining skills. Some sharing of decision making built on a relationship of respect and support is therefore required. This is called 'constructed consent' and appears best in encompassing challenges at the end of life.

The legal position on consent continues to evolve. In the UK the Bolam principle (1957) established the justification for disclosure based on a body of medical opinion. However, this has been increasingly questioned and there is a move towards the balance of power being more with the patient (Marks, 2003). This was first highlighted in the USA (1972) by the case of *Canterbury v Spence*,[10] and this kind of emphasis is now finding its way into common law in England and Wales.[11] In the 1972 case, the right to self-determination for patients was described as the most pre-eminent factor, and was based on the following points.

- Each patient has the right to determine what is done with his or her body.
- Proficiency in diagnosis and therapy is not a full measure of a physician's responsibility; wider skills in communication and decision making need to be recognised.
- It is the prerogative of the patient (not the physician) to determine in which direction his/her interests seem to lie.
- Elucidating the patient's 'perils and options' is prerequisite before obtaining consent.
- The physician's duty to inform is not dependent on the patient's request for disclosure; a physician has a duty to inform when a reasonable patient in the patient's position, if warned of the risk, would be likely to attach significance to it.

Mayberry and Mayberry (2002) studied groups of patients' and lawyers' views on what constituted sufficient information in making a decision about healthcare. Lawyers are known to require more information and, in particular, essential information should include:

- Why is the intervention needed?
- What are the common dangers?
- How is it done?

Bridson *et al.* (2003) call for the recognition of the movement in law from the medical opinion to the reasonable patient. This process needs a change from disclosing information to sharing, and instead of focussing on disclosure, to focus on patient objectives first. In the UK, the Bristol Enquiry (2001) looked at the process of consent leading up to cardiothoracic operations in children, one finding of which was that 'healthcare professionals should adopt the notion of partnership between themselves and the patient, whereby the patient and the professional meet as equals with different expertise'.[12]

The move to a 'reasonable patient' approach to consent helps to overcome the risk of paternalism in decision making.[13] However, faults in this approach also exist. The patient approach is hypothetical and only truly respects patient autonomy when meeting the criteria of a 'typical' patient. What the typical patient would want to know is very much a topic of a debate. This returns to the concept of constructed consent, and the need to understand a patient's approach and values in each case.

Assessment of capacity

Capacity and competency refer to the ability of an individual to make a decision. They are sometimes used interchangeably, although capacity is more commonly referred to in legal judgments.[14] It is essential that all healthcare professionals are confident that their patients have made decisions competently and that a clinician is able to assess this. This section considers the factors important in making assessments of capacity, and in making decisions when the patient lacks capacity.

To have the capacity to make fully informed decisions, a patient should fulfil the following criteria:[15]

- the ability to understand in simple language the purpose of the treatment, its nature, and why it has been proposed
- the ability to understand principal benefits, risks, and alternatives of the intervention
- the ability to understand broadly the consequences of *not* receiving the intervention
- the ability to retain this information and to deliberate on it
- the ability to understand the necessary facts and probabilities
- the ability to make voluntary, uncoerced choice
- the ability to make reasoned choice
- the ability to communicate that choice.

In the UK there is a requirement on the healthcare team to assume that a patient is competent unless proven otherwise, and patients cannot be found lacking in capacity purely on the basis of knowledge or experience, according to GMC (1998) guidelines.

It is unlikely that such strict criteria can be applied to sedation at the end of life. The necessary capacity varies according to the significance of the decision being made, and so a short-acting, light sedative may be requiring of less stringent capacity. For patients with full capacity, decision making with their involvement is relatively straightforward. However, in the periods approaching death it is common for patients to be unable to maintain full capacity.

Factors affecting capacity towards the end of life include:

- spread of disease to brain or meninges
- drug side-effects
- anxiety
- depression
- emotional adjustment to condition
- fears of increased pressure on family and friends.

Health professionals have a responsibility to take every step to try and enhance capacity. This may involve the following:

- adjusting the environment to ensure most effective communication and patient safety
- symptom management
- adjusting medication with euphoric or sedative properties
- treating depression or anxiety
- addressing communication issues.

This raises questions in dealing with patients who may benefit or are benefiting from sedation. Presuming the above steps have been covered, it would be difficult to justify withdrawing sedation or other medication in order to try and achieve increased capacity for consent.

A patient lacking capacity offers a challenge to a healthcare team as to how to approach decision making. In England and Wales, legal responsibility presently lies with the doctor in charge. The British Medical Association (Randall and Downie, 2004: note 59) suggests the following issues are considered when making decisions for patients who lack capacity.

- Liberty – the least restrictive of all options should be employed, with appropriate justification, and enabling maximum enjoyment of life; this would mean using the lowest dose of sedation possible and excluding other treatable conditions.
- Autonomy should be promoted as far as possible, for example by taking into account any advanced statements.
- Dignity should be preserved as far as possible. This would include social and cultural views as well as respect and courtesy. It is debatable as to whether sedation promotes or impairs dignity.
- Patient views should be taken into account as far as possible.

- Privacy – no interventions should be undertaken on sedated patients unless good reasons exist as to why they are needed.
- Health needs should be met as far as resources will allow; this puts a responsibility on professionals to ensure that appropriate interventions are undertaken according to need, even when patients may not be aware.
- Ensure that decisions are free from unfair discrimination.
- Consider the role of proxy decision-makers and those close to the family (discussed in more detail below).
- Consideration is given to a second opinion.
- The multidisciplinary team is involved in any decisions.

Decision making and proxies[16]

In some countries proxy decision-makers are recognised, including much of the rest of Europe and North America. While not yet recognised in England and Wales, it is important to ensure that in theory the following criteria are met (Randall and Downie, 2004: note 59).

- The patient has agreed to the choice and that the proxy is acting on the basis of what the patient would have wanted, and not what they themselves want for the patient.
- The treatment benefits the patient.
- The decision takes into account the patient's wishes.
- The decision takes into account the views of relevant others.
- The decision restricts the freedom of the adult as little as possible.

The risks of using proxy decision-makers include the possibility of disagreement between professionals and proxy, and the balance between respecting an advance directive made by the patient as against a proxy's decision made on the patient's behalf. Even when not nominated formally as proxies, discussions with relatives may be helpful in clarifying what a patient would have wanted. However, both with relatives and, to an extent, with a nominated proxy, the following might arise.

- There is a risk of relatives stating what they would want themselves.
- Relatives' views may well differ from the views of the patient.
- Relatives may not wish to see themselves as the person responsible for withdrawing a treatment or instituting a potentially life-shortening treatment and so may be more proactive.
- A patient's 'off the cuff' remarks may be seen as a genuine wish.
- Conflicts within a family can be hard to resolve and may influence decision making.
- Concerns could occur that decisions are made on motives other than the best interests of the patient.

The pressure on family and proxies in being involved in such decisions is likely to be an issue in the future, and some level of support may well be required during the process of making these decisions.

The role of advance statements[17]

Advance statements regarding treatment decisions are recognised in many countries and can help guide healthcare professionals towards appropriate decision making in cases where patients lack capacity. In relation to sedation at the end of life there may be specific difficulties. For example, it may be very difficult to discuss these issues in advance. To raise sedation at an earlier stage may result in misinterpretation and thus only impair decision making later on. It is not clear whether people can fully comprehend the issues around sedation or know what their experience is going to be. It would be misleading to make advance planning purely regarding sedation, as all possible decisions after the patient loses capacity would need to be included.

The BMA (Randall and Downie, 2004: note 59) questions whether people should be able to decline basic care, defined as interventions with the sole purpose of providing comfort. It could be argued that sedation comes into this category. However, despite these criticisms of specific advance statements, there is a good argument for more patient general wishes or values to be documented in advance. Key considerations for potential patients to reflect on might be:

- the need for comfort and freedom from distress
- the desire to avoid any shortening of life
- the desire to maintain adequate levels of consciousness and clarity of thinking for as long as possible
- the relevance of the views and needs of those close to them, and the effect on them of watching any distress.

Moral and legal justifications for the use of sedation in end-of-life care

The moral arguments around sedation in end-of-life care revolve around reviewing the evidence discussed above, and the use of logical argument and reasoning. First there is the question of the potential harms and benefits from sedation, the relation of these to respect for patient autonomy and how the clinician's beliefs and philosophy of palliative care may affect decision making.

The benefits of sedation lie in the prompt and effective relief of distress from symptoms or from the situation in which a patient now finds him/herself. Being less aware of surroundings and issues may be a benefit to some patients. As time is limited the promptness of the onset of action is particularly important and when life is short there may not be time for more considered or prolonged adjustment of medication or for arranging other interventions.

Conversely, these same benefits could be considered harms for others. Decreased consciousness and the resulting impairment in ability to communicate and be involved in decision making can go greatly against the wishes of some patients. It is impossible to be sure that by decreasing consciousness, and hence awareness of a symptom, the symptom is being treated or that sedation is not merely blunting the usual response to pain and distress. Finally, there is the potential harm of shortening life, although the literature suggests this is an infrequent issue in cases where sedation is used appropriately.

As studies in palliative care studies have shown, professionals may have poor insight into the wishes of patients regarding future treatments (Meystre *et al.*, 1997). Steinhauser (Meystre *et al.*, 1997: note 27) showed that patients did not appreciate losing cognitive ability even for improved symptom control. The risk demonstrated by these findings is that sedation is used through the misperception that it is what the patient wants. This might be partly due to clinicians' values being brought into play, for example, 'I wouldn't want to be left in that state, I'd want to be out of it if I was like that'. But it is also known that patients' views change as they progress through their illness (Slevin *et al.*, 1990), so patients further on in their disease are more likely to take bigger risks and endure greater side-effects for longer life than more healthy individuals. It is also possible to be influenced by the history and founding principles of palliative care, and in particular the 'modern hospice movement'. Here the importance of the mode of death and striving for a peaceful death is usually taught. The use of sedation facilitates a peaceful, distress-free end of life from a professional and family point of view, but this may not be in the best interests of the patients themselves.

This brings one back to the need to respect patient autonomy in decisions over sedation. As previously stated, it is important to accept that there are limitations on patient capacity; nonetheless, when competent, the patient is best placed to weigh up the benefits and harms, and to decide autonomously whether or not sedation is in his/her best interests. To make broad statements about the best action to take in these situations is therefore impossible. The uniqueness of individuals, their circumstances and culture each require careful consideration. The duty on the practising professional is to build a relationship with patients that allows for a mutual understanding of values and approaches to particular situations, and to communicate this in a timely and sensitive manner, if necessary in advance.

Cherny and Portenoy sum up this discussion in the following way: 'Side-effects that impair cognition or run the risk of shortening life become more acceptable when the goals of care of the patient are clearly understood, when the patient's time is limited and when the clinical situation demands an intervention that will have the desired effect in a prompt and effective manner'(Slevin *et al.*, 1990: note 7).

Although the literature suggests there is little effect from sedation on shortening life, there are limitations to some of the published studies. This topic causes concerns for patients, families and professionals, and is worthy of further exploration. The use of sedation requires careful assessment and proportionate treatment, and if professionals feel that they may be shortening life by the use of sedatives, then this may be indication enough for referral to specialist palliative care. It has been estimated that in only two cases out of 238 deaths in a specialist palliative care unit could sedation have contributed significantly to the shortening of patients' lives (Slevin *et al.*, 1990: note 34). The justification for any such consequence lies with the doctrine of double effect (DDE), and the distinction of such actions from either euthanasia or physician-assisted death lies in the intention of the professionals involved.

The doctrine of double effect[18]

The DDE provides a justification for the use of potentially life-shortening interventions at the end of life. Traditionally, this has been associated with morphine use since the ruling involving Dr Adams,[19] a GP accused of causing the death of his patient by using excessive doses of opioids. Lord Devlin, speaking during the case, stated: 'The doctor is entitled to relieve pain and suffering even if the measures he takes may incidentally shorten life'. There is increasing public attention on this area in the UK following a number of high-profile cases. Annie Lindsell, for instance, had motor neurone disease and went to court with the aim of clearing any confusion over the application of the DDE and, in particular, to be sure that any form of distress would be treated under this doctrine and that drugs other than opioids could be used.[20]

The DDE offers a commonsense approach to justify what may intuitively appear to be the right action to take. It helps distinguish between intentional killing and death that is not intended, thus allowing professionals to balance the possible risk of hastening death against benefits to the patient. It has the potential to provide reassurance to the practising healthcare professional, but the criteria are nonetheless open to challenge, and an action that appears intuitively right may not be morally or legally justified. In the United Kingdom the DDE has been recognised in law in the following circumstances (Thorns, 1998).

- The patient must be terminally ill so that it is the illness and not the medication that causes death.
- The treatment must be right and proper as accepted by a responsible body of medical opinion.
- The motivation for the treatment must be to relieve suffering.

When Annie Lindsell applied to the High Court to allow her doctor to use appropriate medication to control her distress, the ruling found that there was no case to answer (Thorns, 1998: note 76).

It would seem wrong to leave a patient distressed for whatever cause. Sedation provides a means of alleviating distress but with risks that may be justified. The intention behind sedation is good – to relieve distress and not to bring about the patient's death; the good effect results from the anxiety-relieving effect of the sedation and not from the death of the patient. Finally, the action appears in proportion to the risk, particularly if a patient is entering the last stages of life. Patients themselves may be able to participate in such discussion, as can be seen in the narrative of some of the scenarios in Part Two. Healthcare professionals can nonetheless be left with the feeling it was their action in giving or prescribing the last injection that caused the death. This is a feeling that may well be uncomfortable for some.

In reality it is hard to know for sure whether it is the injection that causes the ultimate death of a patient, as it must be remembered that symptoms worsen towards the end of life, and increased use of symptomatic treatments is therefore necessary. Death may well have occurred at that time even without intervention. Euthanasia and physician-assisted suicide require an intention on the part of the professional (or some other person) to cause a patient's death, death itself providing relief for the patient's distress. Whilst intention can sometimes be hard to prove, it nonetheless provides a way to distinguish the appropriate use of sedation to relieve distress from forms of assisted dying.

Suggestions for good practice

Having considered the evidence around sedation at the end of life and the moral arguments that surround it, the chapter concludes with a summary of suggestions for good practice. In all decision-making processes the patient's wishes have to be explored to find out to what extent the patient wishes to be involved in current and future treatments, and to what extent relatives or other proxies can be included in the discussions. Similarly, end-of-life decisions require the input of the multidisciplinary team, and the team should ensure that appropriate interventions and support have been offered before sedation is commenced. Sedation should be administered at the lowest dose and for the shortest period in order to gain the desired effect. The use of sedation closer to death is more straightforward to justify.

The final consideration for incompetent patients is the place of routine treatment safeguards that could help prevent abuses of patients in this very vulnerable state. These are a matter of debate and further research, but Cherny and Portenoy (Thorns, 1998: note 34) have put forward a number of suggested safeguards:

- both patient and family wish for sedation rather than endurance of symptoms and are fully involved in decision making
- the decision is made rationally, voluntarily and consistently
- the intention of all should be the relief of symptoms and not to shorten a patient's life (which comes under the doctrine of double effect)
- diagnostic and prognostic clarity should be established
- use of a second opinion
- explicit processes for documentation and review
- the symptom being refractory.

Additional points that could be added to this list are:

- benchmarking against others' practice
- regular training to ensure effective steps are taken to treat any reversible conditions before commencing sedation
- protocols for the initiation of sedation.

Suggestions for future research and development

Future research in this area needs to focus on:

- exploration of the knowledge and perceptions of patients, families and professionals regarding sedation at the end of life across different cultures
- exploration of how people make decisions and express their preferences, especially across different cultures and with the advent of a more choice-dominated approach to healthcare

- individualised assessment on patients' information and decision-making needs and preferences, raising the possibility of setting standards for information giving regarding sedation
- general methods of improving patient-centred decision making, especially in cases where patient capacity is poor
- developing suitable methods of assessing capacity in a palliative care population
- exploring the role and effect of advance directives and proxies in end-of-life decision making.

Short cases

Short case 1

John has a carcinoma of his mouth, which has spread extensively over the left side of his face. This causes him severe pain both from the tumour itself as well as resulting neuropathic pain from local damage to nerves. Conventional analgesia has only been partly successful, there are no oncological interventions available to him, and the chronic pain specialists have been unable to offer any helpful interventions. Swallowing is becoming difficult as a result of the tumour and John wishes that his life was 'all over'.

The team looking after John's care recommend a syringe driver with midazolam to relieve his distress from both the pain and his general distress. John becomes drowsy, he can still wake and talk for brief periods of time but is mainly asleep. A decision against artificial feeding and hydration has already been made with John and he dies a week later.

Short case 2

Mary has motor neurone disease (MND); in time she will become unable to use her arms or legs, to swallow or to speak. Currently she is able to sit in a wheelchair and communicate. She can take some things by mouth but her intake needs topping up via a feeding tube into her stomach. She is desperately frightened by the thought of what will happen to her in the future. She has asked for her life to be ended but understands this is not legal. Instead she is asking to be sedated to relieve her distress. She appreciates this may shorten her life but is happy for this to happen. The team have tried hard to resolve Mary's fears but without success. They are reluctant to provide long-term deep sedation because of the likely shortening of Mary's life. Instead they offer short-term light sedation with a view to breaking the cycle of Mary's fear and helping to maintain her trust by partially acceding to her request.

Short case 3[21]

Gill is a 70-year-old lady with cancer of the lung and a previous history of schizophrenia. She develops delusions and progressive agitation which does not respond to 12 mg of haloperidol. Over the next 24 hours she receives 325 mg of levomepromazine and 60 mg of midazolam. Her breathing changes and she appears to be developing excess secretions on her chest. The agitation remains and she is given phenobarbitone 200 mg. She dies six hours later.

Notes to Chapter 6

[1] A definition of the meaning and use of this term follows shortly.

[2] Tables reprinted with permission from Elsevier, Sykes NP and Thorns A (2003a) The use of opioids and sedatives at the end of life in palliative care. *Lancet Oncol.* **4**: 312–18.

[3] *Ibid.* Note 9,

[4] *Ibid.* Note 12.

[5] *Ibid.* Note 11.

[6] Some short cases have been included at the end of this chapter to illustrate various uses of sedation.

[7] *See* Chapter 5.

[8] Quill *et al.* (1997); Morita *et al.* (1999) (especially note 7).

[9] The exact content of this discussion depends on the physician's judgment.

[10] *Canterbury v. Spence* (1972) 464 F2d 772 (DC, 1972) USA.

[11] Cf. *Bolitho v. City & Hackney Health Authority* (1997) All ER 771 and (1998) All AC 232.

[12] Bristol Royal Infirmary Inquiry (2001).

[13] Cf. *Pearce v United Bristol Healthcare NHS Trust* (1999) 48 BMLR 118, a common law decision that led to a change of direction towards the reasonable patient standard, as opposed to the reasonable body of professional opinion that has prevailed since the time of Bolam (i.e. 1957).

[14] British Medical Association (2003). An alternative (more semantically accurate) interpretation is that capacity is that which you measure in order to determine competency. The difficulty using the term 'competency' is with its opposite, so it is falling out of favour. Incompetence has unwanted connotations, whereas incapacity does not.

[15] General Medical Council (1998); Randall and Downie (2004), especially note 59.

[16] *See* Chapter 3.

[17] *See* Chapter 4.

[18] *See* Chapter 4.

[19] *R v. Adams* (1957) Crim Law Rev. 365.

[20] Dyer C Dr (1997) Terminally ill woman in 'painless death' plea. *The Guardian.* October 29.

[21] Short case 3 appeared in Sykes NP and Thorns A (2003b) Sedative use in the last week of life and the implications for end of life decision-making. *Arch Intern Med.* **163**: 341–4. Reprinted with permission. Copyrighted © 2003, American Medical Association. All rights reserved.

Part Two

Case histories and clinical scenarios

The following histories are drawn from real life. Names have been changed and details altered in order to protect the identity of former patients, and to show respect for the confidentiality of the families concerned. Each case consists of first an abstract and then an outline of how the case was managed, including a description of complicating factors and comments detailing clinicians' perspectives. Separate notes have been added at the end that focus on the ethical implications of each case.

Case history 1: Alan Adair

Abstract
Mr Adair is a 53-year-old man with widespread lung cancer who becomes dependent on a ventilator after undergoing a lung biopsy. His family is initially reluctant for him to be informed of the severity of his condition. After he is informed about his diagnosis and prognosis he decides that he wishes all active interventions to be stopped and to be sedated.

Case history
Mr Alan Adair was a 53-year-old photographer. He had smoked 20 cigarettes a day since the age of 16. Initially he developed a cough productive of yellow sputum, and he visited his GP who prescribed a course of amoxicillin (an antibiotic). However, despite an initial improvement in his cough, his symptoms persisted. In addition he noted that he was losing his appetite and his wife remarked that he appeared to be losing weight. Mr Adair refused to return to his GP as he felt that 'everything would be fine'.

Clinician's thoughts: Mr Adair, in common with many men, is reluctant to consult medical services.

Three weeks later he still had a productive cough and had now developed a high temperature and taken to his bed. His wife called out the GP who arranged for admission to the local hospital for treatment of suspected pneumonia. On admission to the hospital Mr Adair was found to have multiple problems. He had symptoms and signs of bilateral pleural effusions (fluid around the lungs), he had evidence of pneumonia, his chest x-ray also showed multiple nodules throughout both lungs (suggestive of secondary cancer) and erosion of one of his ribs (also likely to be due to secondary cancer). He had a mildly elevated serum calcium and was anaemic.

Clinician's thoughts: Mr Adair has symptoms and signs in keeping with widespread

lung cancer. He also has pneumonia. Although the investigations are highly sugges-
tive of cancer, without a biopsy it is not possible to be categorical about his diagnosis.
It is possible that Mr Adair, himself, suspected that he had underlying cancer and
that this is why he was reluctant to consult his doctor.

He was started on intravenous antibiotics and a few days later the pleural
effusion was drained and sent for analysis. No malignant cells were identified, although the protein content of the fluid was highly suggestive of
malignancy.

Clinician's thoughts: The evidence in favour of a cancer diagnosis is mounting but
is still not conclusive. Without a definitive diagnosis it is not possible for the clini-
cian to recommend treatment. This can mean that some patients are subjected to
multiple invasive tests and biopsies to determine the underlying disorder only then
to discover that the diagnosis is widespread (incurable) cancer. Other patients never
receive a definitive diagnosis at all.

Although there was a slight improvement in Mr Adair's condition with the
intravenous antibiotics, he remained generally quite frail. There was a
strong suspicion that Mr Adair had an underlying malignancy but there
was still no tissue diagnosis. The following day he had a bronchoscopy (an
investigation with a flexible tube inserted into the lungs) to obtain a
biopsy for analysis. Unfortunately, Mr Adair did not make a good recovery
from the procedure.[1] His breathing rapidly deteriorated and he had to be
intubated (have a tube placed down his throat into his lungs to help him
breathe). He was then transferred to the intensive therapy unit (ITU).

Clinician's thoughts: Every procedure carries a risk of complications. It is the
responsibility of medical staff to obtain informed consent prior to undertaking any
invasive procedure. The low risk of requiring ventilation may or may not have been
communicated to Mr Adair; in either event it is likely that he would still have
agreed to the procedure because it was recommended to him by his doctors.
Although clinicians are becoming better at explaining the risks of procedures, it is
not always clear that they adequately explain the expected benefits. It may, for
instance, have been the case that Mr Adair was told that the bronchoscopy was
necessary 'so we can find out what is wrong with you'. In which case he would
almost certainly have agreed to the procedure. But his response may have been
different if the clinician had said 'We are very suspicious that you have widespread
lung cancer but we cannot be absolutely certain without a biopsy. If the biopsy does
confirm cancer then we will have very little to offer you in terms of treatment.
Would you still like to have the biopsy?'[2]

After a few days on the ITU the biopsy result confirmed the diagnosis of
lung cancer and Mr Adair was referred to the oncology team. In the meantime, several attempts were made to wean Mr Adair off the ventilator but
without success. A tracheostomy was performed and Mr Adair's sedation
was then lightened.

Clinician's thoughts: After thorough investigation, Mr Adair is confirmed as having
lung cancer with secondary spread. Unfortunately his poor underlying lung func-
tion means that he has now become dependent on the ventilator.

The oncologists reviewed Mr Adair's case and felt that given the widespread nature of his disease and his poor general health he would not benefit from chemotherapy or any other anti-cancer intervention. The biopsy results and the opinion of the oncologists were explained to Mr Adair's wife, who was obviously greatly distressed by this news. Mr Adair was referred to the hospital palliative care team for advice about ongoing management.

The ITU ward staff had explained to Mrs Adair that it was important for her husband to be informed of his diagnosis and likely prognosis so that he could make informed decisions about his future care. Mrs Adair was unhappy with this approach and felt that it was unfair to burden him with such information. However, ITU staff were quite clear that concealing information from Mr Adair was not an option. An appointment was made for Mrs Adair to be present the following day when a senior member of the ITU staff was due to speak with Mr Adair about his prognosis and diagnosis.[3]

Clinician's thoughts: Mrs Adair was given the information about her husband's diagnosis when he was still unconscious, and the ITU staff were unsure whether he would survive the next few days. If he had been awake and alert at the time then the staff would probably have communicated the information to him directly. Unfortunately tensions often arise when relatives are given information about diagnosis/prognosis before (or instead of) patients themselves.

The following day Mrs Adair arrived on the ward and immediately went in to visit her husband. She decided to tell him the 'bad news' herself rather than wait for the consultant to arrive. She informed him that he had 'terminal cancer' and that 'nothing more could be done to help him'.

Clinician's thoughts: The ITU staff were concerned about how Mrs Adair had communicated the diagnosis/prognosis to her husband. They were worried that she may have been 'too blunt' and had 'painted it blacker than it really was'. There is no doubt that trained nursing or medical staff would have communicated the information in a different manner. Nonetheless, Mrs Adair felt that it was her responsibility to speak to her husband directly about this matter, and it is not at all clear that professional staff would have done a better job.

At this point the palliative care team arrived on the ward. The ITU staff explained to the palliative care team that they wanted advice on the management of the terminal phase of this gentleman after withdrawal of ventilatory support. The plan was to stop the artificial ventilation and to provide adequate pain relief and sedation during the terminal phase.

Clinician's thoughts: It became apparent to the palliative care team that the plan had not yet been discussed with the patient or his family. The team therefore offered to facilitate discussion of the issues surrounding end-of-life care with the patient and his family.[4]

The ITU consultant, the palliative care doctor, the ITU nurse and Mrs Adair then spoke with Mr Adair.[5] Mr Adair was unable to speak clearly because of the tracheostomy but was able to communicate with nods and shakes of his head and with the use of lip-reading. It was explained to Mr Adair that his cancer was no longer amenable to anti-cancer therapy and that because of the poor condition of his lungs he was now dependent on the ventilator. Mr Adair indicated that he understood all of this and that his only wish was to go home.

Clinician's thoughts: Unfortunately discharge home while still on a ventilator was not a very practical prospect.

A discussion then ensued relating to withdrawal of ventilation. It was explained to Mr Adair that if the ventilation was reduced or stopped then he would most likely become increasingly confused and drowsy and would lapse into a coma and die. Mr Adair indicated that he was keen to stop all active treatments, and that he wished to be disconnected from as much machinery as possible. At this stage he was being nasogastrically fed (a tube inserted up his nose into his stomach), he was on a ventilator, he had a tracheostomy (a breathing hole in his throat) and he was on continuous intravenous fluid plus other intravenous drug infusions. He was also having continuous measurement of oxygen saturations, ECG, temperature, pulse and blood pressure.

Clinician's thoughts: For many patients with cancer the decision to stop 'active treatment' does not have any immediate consequences. If a patient with progressive disease elects not to have any further chemotherapy then the patient may still live for many weeks or months before any further deterioration and eventual death. Mr Adair's decision to stop active treatment, on the other hand, was likely to have far more immediate effects. He was receiving intensive life support and a decision to stop treatment could rapidly result in his death. For this reason, the palliative care team felt it was important that Mr Adair fully understood the consequences of his decisions.

Mr Adair explained to the ITU staff that he wished to see his family. He indicated that he wanted the ventilation to be withdrawn after he had seen his family, and under cover of appropriate sedation. He declined the offer of a visit from a spiritual advisor.

Clinician's thoughts: Mr Adair realised that withdrawal of treatment would probably rapidly result in his death. He wished to 'say his goodbyes' to his family, and requested that he be sufficiently sedated so that he did not experience any distress when his ventilation was withdrawn. Mr Adair was asked whether or not he considered himself to be a 'spiritual' or a 'religious person'. His medical records noted that he was 'Church of England'. However, on direct questioning Mr Adair reported that although he was baptised an Anglican he had never been a 'churchgoer' and did not really believe in 'organised religion'. (He did, however, feel that there was a 'higher purpose' to the universe and that there may be some existence beyond death.)[6]

At this point there was a change in nursing shift. Due to poor communication and handover, the new ITU nurse proceeded to commence a propofol infusion (a general anaesthetic) on Mr Adair, because he was agitated and was requesting some sedation. This was not in accordance with the previously agreed plan, which had been to provide him with small doses of midazolam (a milder sedative) as and when required, in order to manage any anxiety or distress until after he had seen his family, but before ventilation was withdrawn. Shortly after starting the propofol infusion Mr Adair was rendered unresponsive.[7]

Clinician's thoughts: Things do not always proceed according to plan.

Shortly after the propofol infusion had been started, Mr Adair's wife, brother, and two daughters arrived on the ward (as previously agreed) to say their goodbyes. The ITU consultant explained that the sedation could be quite quickly reversed and Mr Adair would soon wake up again. However, Mrs Adair was now keen that the sedation should not be reduced since she was relieved to see her husband looking so peaceful. She felt that were he to be woken from his sedation to see his family surrounding him at his bedside, it would be likely to cause him undue distress.

Clinician's thoughts: Although the original plan had been for Mr Adair to see his family and then be sedated, unforeseen events had resulted in the sedation occurring prematurely. Prior to this heavy sedation Mr Adair had understandably been quite agitated and distressed about his condition. Mrs Adair clearly had her husband's best interests at heart and did not wish to see him suffer any further distress. However, the palliative care team felt that since Mr Adair had been competent at the time when his request was made, it should be honoured.[8]

During discussions with the family it was explained that Mr Adair had clearly stated his wish not to be heavily sedated until after he had seen his family. It was therefore agreed that the sedation should be lightened. It was explained that this would also provide Mr Adair with another opportunity to discuss his future management, in case he had changed his mind about withdrawal of treatment.

After a tearful family reunion Mr Adair indicated that he now wished to be disconnected from as much machinery as was possible. He was initially started on a subcutaneous midazolam infusion (at a rate of 30 mg per 24 hours), and in addition he was given diamorphine (10 mg per 24 hours). The intention of this treatment was to provide some level of sedation and pain relief, but not to render him as heavily sedated as the propofol infusion had done previously. It was explained to Mr Adair that if he managed to establish spontaneous respiration without the use of the ventilator, every effort would be made to respect his wish to be discharged home.

Clinician's thoughts: The palliative care team had promised Mr Adair that he would be adequately sedated in order to prevent distress arising from discontinuation of ventilation. However, the team did not wish to sedate him so heavily that they brought about his premature death due to respiratory arrest. The intention of the sedation was symptom relief and not hastening death.[9]

Over the next 12 hours Mr Adair required one further increase in mida-zolam dosage. By 6am the following morning he was being maintained on midazolam (60 mg) and diamorphine (10 mg over 24 hours). At this point the ventilation was gradually withdrawn without undue distress to Mr Adair. He survived for six hours after withdrawal of all artificial ventila-tion but did not regain consciousness prior to death.[10]

Case history 2: David Deakin

Abstract
David Deakin is a 61-year-old man with terminal metastatic colon cancer. His daughter is his main carer. Mr Deakin tends to devolve all decision making to his daughter, Karen. This can cause some tension with the medical and nursing staff, who feel that Karen has unrealistic expectations about her father's prognosis. The staff feels that she is 'interfering' with the appropriate management of Mr Deakin's symptoms. The conflict reaches a crisis as Mr Deakin's condition deteriorates and Karen asks the medical team to stop administering morphine. The clinical team feel that the morphine is providing symptomatic relief, but Karen feels that it is causing unacceptable side-effects.

Case history
Mr David Deakin is a 61-year-old school caretaker. He originally presented two years previously with malignant melanoma (skin cancer) which was treated by surgery. Following his initial treatment he was disease free for 18 months. Six months ago the cancer was found to have spread to his liver and he was started on palliative chemotherapy. After four cycles of treatment he was restaged and found to have progressive disease (locally recurrent disease, ascites, worsening liver metastases, lung metastases and malignant pleural effusions). Currently, his main complaints are of breathlessness, insomnia, a feeling of abdominal fullness, and general immobility. He has a past medical history of chronic obstructive airways disease and heart failure, for which he is receiving maximum medical therapy. He is also morbidly obese (body mass index greater than 35). He has been a widower for five years. He has three adult children (one daughter and two sons). Both sons are in regular telephone contact, but are not involved in his day-to-day care. His unmarried daughter lives at home and is his main carer.

Clinician's thoughts: Mr Deakin now has widespread and progressive malignant disease. He has a poor prognosis. His principal symptom is breathlessness. He has many possible causes for this symptom including pleural effusions (fluid around the lungs), ascites (fluid in the abdomen which can cause splinting of the diaphragm), chronic obstructive airways disease (chronic bronchitis and emphysema), heart failure and morbid obesity. Although he has three children it is only his daughter who visits regularly.[11]

David is initially referred to the palliative care team for help with symptom control and for 'psycho-social' support. His breathlessness (which is his chief complaint) is thought to be due to a combination of factors. He has a left-sided pleural effusion, which has been drained on two previous occasions. A recent ultrasound scan has revealed a moderately sized, loculated, left pleural effusion with no obvious site for further drainage. The scan also confirms the presence of a small amount of ascites. He has undergone several previous paracenteses (procedures to drain the abdominal fluid) with little symptomatic improvement. The most recent attempt resulted in a 'dry tap'.

Clinician's thoughts: There are no easily reversible causes for his breathlessness.[12]

The medical and nursing staff on the ward are particularly concerned about the way in which Mr Deakin's daughter (Karen) is coping with her father's illness. During the most recent admission Karen has been living permanently in the hospital. Despite being fully informed about her father's poor prognosis and the extent of his disease, she seems unable to accept that no further active intervention will be helpful.

The palliative care team assess Mr Deakin and his daughter. They identify that the major physical complaint is of breathlessness associated with some anxiety. David had previously tried diazepam for these problems and the nursing staff felt that this had proved to be of some symptomatic benefit. However, Karen became quite upset when her father became drowsier and she did not wish for this treatment to be continued. The medical team then stopped administering diazepam.[13]

Clinician's thoughts: Diazepam is an anxiolytic and can be helpful for patients who have a degree of anxiety or panic associated with their breathlessness. It can cause some sedation (indeed, that is probably the mechanism by which it relieves breathlessness). The diazepam had been tried (and stopped) by the medical team before the patient was referred to the palliative care team. Karen was quite clear that she did not wish her father to receive this drug again because of the perceived side-effects.[14]

The other issue identified by the palliative care team was related to communication between the patient, his daughter and the multi-professional team. By mutual agreement Mr Deakin was never seen in the absence of his daughter. However, he tended not to answer direct questions from the medical or nursing staff and left most decisions to his daughter. He would occasionally respond to questions with just one- or two-word answers.

Karen often asked exactly the same question of different members of the multi-professional team. This occasionally resulted in tensions within the team, and between the team and Karen. The team felt that Karen was 'checking up' on them and that she did not trust their judgment. They felt that if she asked a question and did not get the answer that she wanted to hear from one member of staff, she would keep asking until she found someone who gave her the 'right' answer. This was particularly the case when Karen sought reassurance about her father's prognosis. Occasionally, some members of the multi-professional team would respond to questions about David's prognosis with a slightly more optimistic response than other members of the team. Karen was quick to pick up any discrepancies in the answers she received and would constantly challenge staff members with slightly conflicting comments made by their colleagues. Despite repeated explanations relating to the terminal nature of her father's condition, Karen was reluctant to accept that nothing further could be done to prolong her father's survival.

Clinician's thoughts: This case illustrates two common problems. Firstly there is the issue of assessing Mr Deakin's wishes. Karen always insisted on being present when staff were communicating with her father, and he agreed to this arrangement. On one occasion he was asked if he would like Karen to leave while he was spoken to privately, but he declined the offer. However, the staff found the arrangement to be very frustrating – they sometimes felt that Karen was 'projecting' her own thoughts, fears and worries onto her father. For instance, the nurses did not feel that Mr Deakin himself had been particularly concerned by the drowsiness associated with using diazepam, but they felt that he had been pressurised into refusing this drug by his daughter.

Secondly, there is the issue of communication within a large multi-professional team.[15] By asking the same questions of enough individuals, Karen was able to detect slight differences in their answers. Karen interpreted this as either reflecting ignorance on behalf of the staff or as a deliberate act of concealment. When patients or relatives ask about prognoses there are quite likely to be discrepancies between the answers that they receive, both because of genuine uncertainty and because some professionals find it too difficult or uncomfortable to be completely frank in their responses.[16]

On the advice of the palliative care team Mr Deakin was started on buspirone for the management of both anxiety and breathlessness. It was also suggested that Karen and/or her father might like to speak to the oncology counsellor to discuss any worries or concerns they had about the treatment. A discussion within the multidisciplinary team reinforced the importance of the staff providing the Deakin family with consistent, clear and unambiguous information and avoiding the temptation to agree with any over-optimistic assessments made by Karen.

Clinician's thoughts: Buspirone is an anxiolytic which has also been shown in a few studies to have some effects on relieving breathlessness. It was selected by the palliative care team in this instance because of its beneficial effects on anxiety, and because Karen was very reluctant to consider morphine (usually the drug of first choice for the palliation of breathlessness). Because of Karen's forceful personality and because of previous conflict with the clinical staff, the palliative care team was wary of provoking any further confrontation.

Four days after starting buspirone there did appear to be a mild symptomatic improvement in Mr Deakin's dyspnoea. However, Karen approached the medical team and requested that the buspirone be stopped because she was concerned about potential side-effects. She had read in a textbook that buspirone can result in palpitations, chest pain and drowsiness, and she felt unhappy about her father continuing with this medication. When Mr Deakin was approached to discuss the issue his daughter answered all of the questions on his behalf. The nurses felt quite unhappy about stopping the buspirone, as they felt that it was contributing to the patient's comfort. Moreover, there were some concerns that Karen's views should not be taken to reflect the views of her father. The palliative care team was asked for advice on the best way to proceed.

Clinician's thoughts: This represents a difficult problem and illustrates well the difference between the 'ideal' world and the messy reality of practical ethics. Palliative care philosophy places a high regard on patient autonomy and expects patients to take responsibility for making decisions about their own healthcare. Teams strive to respect those decisions even when they do not accord with their own, or even if they do not seem to be in a patient's best interests. Indeed, team members often act as patient's advocate when patients say they wish to 'stop treatment' but don't wish to 'upset the doctor'. However, in this circumstance, the decision of the patient to devolve autonomy to his daughter was not accepted easily by the clinical staff.

Palliative care teams are often faced with situations where patients themselves refuse treatments that the team believes are helpful. If Mr Deakin had clearly articulated that he did not wish to continue buspirone for whatever reason, it would have been quickly accepted by the staff. However, he did not do that; instead he reacted ambivalently. The staff's perception was that if he had been seen alone and asked whether or not he wanted to continue with the drug, he would have agreed to do so.

The situation was further complicated by the fact that buspirone is not a first-choice drug to manage breathlessness, which meant that it was difficult to persuade Karen (and thus her father) that it was unreasonable to insist on stopping it.

After long discussions with Karen (in the presence of her father) it was agreed that the buspirone should stop. However, it was recognised that breathlessness was a significant symptom, and so it was agreed that Mr Deakin should have a trial of oral morphine. His medication was therefore changed to *as required* oral morphine. Once again the nurses reported that the morphine appeared to provide some symptomatic benefit. Mr Deakin was becoming increasingly distressed with his general condition, and he was often found to be calling out in the middle of the night for help.

By this stage he was unable to articulate exactly what his distress related to, but the nurses noted that once he was given the oral morphine he tended to settle. Nonetheless, after two or three days of this treatment Karen once again objected to the medical staff, this time about perceived side-effects of the oral morphine. In particular, she felt that the oral morphine was making her father unacceptably drowsy. The nursing staff concurred that the morphine was indeed causing some drowsiness but felt that the benefits of the morphine outweighed the side-effects.[17] By this stage Mr Deakin was having difficulty taking oral medication and it was necessary for the morphine to be administered by intermittent or continuous subcutaneous administration. Once again, whenever the medical staff tried to ascertain Mr Deakin's views directly their questions were answered by Karen.

Clinician's thoughts: By this stage it was difficult to know whether or not Mr Deakin was still competent. He was still awake and conscious but not answering questions. His condition was deteriorating and it was expected that he would die within the next few days or small number of weeks. In England, in an incompetent patient, there is no legal duty to act in accordance with the wishes of the next of kin. Medical staff are required to act in the 'best interests' of the patient. However, it was clear that up until this point, the staff had been accepting (albeit reluctantly) that Karen was able to make decisions on behalf of her father because he had willingly delegated that responsibility. It was therefore difficult to now act contrary to her wishes. Nonetheless, the palliative care team took the view that since their primary responsibility lay with caring for Mr Deakin, it was their duty to make sure that he was kept comfortable.

(It is interesting to consider whether the team would have acted any differently if Karen had not been involved, and if Mr Deakin (when competent) had refused opiates,[18] i.e. would the team have felt justified in giving them to him when he became incompetent as his condition deteriorated?)[19]

Mr Deakin was started on a continuous subcutaneous infusion of diamorphine. He appeared to become more settled and he died peacefully six days later. His daughter was never fully reconciled to the decision. Although she accepted that the ultimate cause of her father's death was metastatic cancer, she blamed his final deterioration on the use of opiates.[20]

Case history 3: Eric Evans

Abstract

Eric Evans is a 94-year-old man with brain metastases from a colonic primary. There is disagreement about the most appropriate way to manage his condition. Eventually Mr Evans agrees to aggressive treatment with neurosurgery and laparotomy. However, he never fully recovers from the surgery and despite being disease free requests that active treatment is stopped.

Case history

Mr Eric Evans was a 94-year-old man who presented to the casualty department following a collapse at home. He gave a history of becoming increasingly unwell over the previous three months. He had been losing some weight and had noticed an alteration in his bowel habit. On examination he was found to have a mild left-sided hemiplegia. He was therefore admitted to the medical ward. Mr Evans had been a widower for 20 years. He had one remaining son, aged 69, who lived approximately 100 miles away. Mr Evans lived alone and up until this admission had been self-caring.

During his admission to hospital he underwent a CT brain scan which revealed a solitary right frontal brain metastasis (secondary cancer). Subsequent investigation confirmed the source of the primary as a colonic carcinoma. Mr Evans was referred to the medical oncologist for an opinion. The medical oncologist, Dr Peck, felt that the most appropriate treatment for Mr Evans would be palliative cranial radiotherapy. He did not feel that Mr Evans was fit enough to tolerate systemic chemotherapy.

Mr Evans was therefore referred to the clinical oncologist, Dr Hadley, who felt that more aggressive management was warranted. She was of the opinion that Mr Evans should have a surgical excision of his solitary brain metastasis, followed by a resection of his primary tumour. This would then be followed by adjuvant radiotherapy.[21] Dr Hadley was concerned that just because Mr Evans was 94 years old, he should not be 'written off'.

*Clinician's comments: Mr Evans' prognosis is poor and the **medical** oncologist, Dr Peck, felt that palliative treatment was most appropriate. However, the **clinical** oncologist, Dr Hadley, felt that more aggressive management was warranted and she was concerned that Mr Evans was being discriminated against because of his age.[22] Dr Peck, on the other hand, was of the view that Mr Evans' prognosis was extremely poor, that the likelihood of successfully treating the tumour with surgery was very low, and that his advanced years would make the probability of successful treatment even lower. Dr Hadley argued that although the chance of success was low it was 'the only chance of success'.[23] This case illustrates the difficulties that can occur when clinicians cannot agree on what is the best or most appropriate management of a condition. Both Dr Hadley and Dr Peck agreed that the chances of successful treatment were extremely low; Dr Hadley simply felt that aggressive management was warranted whereas Dr Peck did not.*

There was considerable concern expressed by nursing staff on the ward that Mr Evans was being encouraged to accept a treatment he did not really want. They felt that the surgery had been presented to both the patient and his son as the only chance of 'cure', and that other alternatives (such as more conservative or palliative approaches) had not been adequately discussed.[24]

Clinician's comments: How information is presented to patients can have a dramatic effect on whether or not they will consent to a procedure. It is much less likely that Mr Evans would have agreed to surgery if Dr Hadley had said, 'I'm afraid that you have widespread cancer, and although it may be technically possible to remove all of the tumour with surgery, this will be a very extensive procedure with a high risk of complications and a low chance of success – your quality of life may be better preserved by a more conservative approach, although there is no chance that this latter approach will get rid of all the cancer'. Dr Hadley was quite clear in her own mind that surgery was the appropriate treatment for Mr Evans, and so she had set out to try and persuade him to agree to active treatment. Indeed, Dr Hadley felt that it would be unethical not to try to persuade Mr Evans to have surgery, since she felt that this was in his best interests.[25]

Eventually Mr Evans agreed to sign the consent form for cranial surgery to remove his brain metastasis. He was therefore transferred to a specialist neurosurgery centre for cranial surgery. Two weeks later he was readmitted to the ward following a 'successful' excision of a solitary brain metastasis, which was confirmed to be metastatic adenocarcinoma of the colon. There was no noticeable improvement in his left-sided weakness following the surgery. Shortly after arrival on the ward, Mr Evans was assessed by the general surgeons with a view to undertaking bowel surgery for resection of his primary tumour. He had previously been seen by the surgeons at the time of his original diagnosis. At that stage the surgeons had declined to operate as they did not feel that he would benefit from surgery. However, they were now presented with a patient who had undergone a resection of a solitary brain metastasis with the expectation that definitive surgery to his primary tumour would be undertaken thereafter.

Clinician's comments: Events now seem to be moving under their own momentum. Although the general surgeon was originally not very keen to operate on Mr Evans' primary cancer, he feels that it may now be appropriate to do so because Mr Evans has already had his brain metastasis removed. If the primary tumour is not now resected then there would have been limited value in undergoing surgery for the brain metastasis.

By this stage Mr Evans had become quite withdrawn and seemed rather depressed. He did, however, agree to undergo the bowel surgery. His son remained keen for active intervention, particularly as he felt that this was the only way that his father's life could be saved.[26] Mr Evans' bowel surgery was 'successful' in that his tumour was completely resected. However, post-operatively he failed to thrive. He was reviewed by the palliative care team three days after his operation. At this stage he was very withdrawn, he was bed-bound and not eating; he had a central venous line *in situ*, and he was on intravenous antibiotics. He was difficult to engage in conversation but did indicate that he was in some discomfort. He also said he was 'fed up' and wanted to be left alone. He was started on some regular analgesia (paracetamol 1 gram qds). Over the following 10 days there was very little change in his condition. He remained extremely withdrawn and reluctant to engage with staff. He complained of 'aching all over' although could not specify any site in particular. His analgesics had by this stage been increased to regular co-codamol (two tablets, four times a day).

Clinician's comments: Both the neurosurgery and the bowel surgery have been 'successful' and Mr Evans is ostensibly disease free (although with a high chance of developing recurrent disease). However, the trauma of two major operations within a month in a 94-year-old man resulted in considerable morbidity.

Eleven days after surgery he was reviewed again by the palliative care team. At this stage he was looking extremely frail and withdrawn, and remained bed-bound. He refused to open his eyes when speaking. When he was asked by the consultant in palliative care how he was feeling, he said 'Just leave me alone. I would be happy to go. Stop pulling me about. I've had a good life, I've lived for 90 years or more and I've had enough. Why are you doing this to me?'. The palliative care consultant responded by asking Mr Evans if he wanted all of his treatment to stop. Mr Evans replied that he did. It was explained to him that stopping his antibiotics and fluids may result in his premature death. Mr Evans said that he realised this but still wanted all of his treatment to stop.[27]

The palliative care consultant sympathised with Mr Evans' request and said that he would speak with the surgeon in charge and convey to him Mr Evans' wishes. However, it was highly likely that the surgeon would wish to hear Mr Evans' wishes directly. At this point Mr Evans simply responded, 'Why does nobody listen to anything I say? I've been asking people for days to stop pulling me about, but nobody ever listens'.

Clinician's comments: Mr Evans is finding the burden of continued treatment to be intolerable. He wishes to stop. It is possible that he is depressed, although on direct questioning he denies that this is the case – it is simply that he is angry and fed up with his continued ill health. Even if he were depressed he may still be able to make a competent decision to refuse treatment.[28] Mr Evans was able to retain, process and weigh the relevant information about his condition and he came to a competent decision to stop treatment. However, in view of the intensive treatment that he had already undergone, and in anticipation of disagreement about his competence to refuse further treatment, the palliative care team felt it would be prudent to obtain a second opinion as regards Mr Evans' competency.[29]

Later that day the surgical consultant reviewed whether Mr Evans was making a competent decision to stop active treatment. He agreed that Mr Evans was competent to refuse further treatment, and at that point the antibiotics were stopped and the central venous line removed.

Clinician's comments: It may well have been sensible to obtain a psychiatric opinion about Mr Evans' competency. However, under English law it is not necessary to do so. The Department of Health has issued guidelines on determining competency, and these do not require that a psychiatrist be involved in the assessment.[30] However, in this case, as there was the possibility of a co-morbid psychiatric disorder (depression) it may well have been wise to do so.

Dr Hadley felt that it was unacceptable to withdraw treatment from Mr Evans despite acknowledging that this was the patient's clearly stated wish. She felt that having put him through all of the previous surgery, 'We owe it to him to make him get better'.[31] She felt that the medical and nursing staff had a duty to persuade Mr Evans to continue with his treatment and that his decision to stop treatment should not be taken at its face value.[32]

Clinician's comments: Dr Hadley feels that there is no ethical obligation to respect Mr Evans' wishes to stop treatment. She feels that were he to recover from further surgery he would be grateful that the medical staff had not 'given up' on him. Furthermore, there seems to be a feeling that because Mr Evans had already undergone so much medical and surgical treatment, there was a greater obligation to continue active treatment than if he had never agreed to treatment in the first place.[33]

Despite Dr Hadley's objections, no change was made to Mr Evans' management. The following day he was transferred to the local hospice for continuing care and died peacefully 24 hours later.

Case history 4: Guy Gifford

Abstract
Mr Gifford is a 52-year-old man with widespread lung cancer. He is admitted to hospital because of severe pain. There is disagreement between Mr Gifford and the clinical team about the appropriateness of administering cardiopulmonary resuscitation. He is transferred to the hospice where his pain can only be controlled by escalating the dose of opiates to the point where Mr Gifford becomes deeply sedated.

Case history
Mr Guy Gifford was a 52-year-old baker. He had been suffering from metastatic small cell carcinoma of the lung for one year. He now had metastases in the brain, lung, liver and bones. Mr Gifford had a long-term partner who was 15 years younger than himself. Together they had had two daughters aged 13 and 16. His partner was fully aware of the extent of his disease, and although his children had been informed that he had cancer, it was not clear that they understood the severity of his condition.

He was admitted to hospital for the management of severe pain in the thoracic spine. The pain was secondary to metastatic disease at this site, which had previously been irradiated. He had recently completed a course of chemotherapy, and treatment had been stopped because of progressive disease. Mr Gifford was keen on pursuing further active treatment; however, the oncologist told him, 'You are not fit enough at the moment...but if your condition improves then we may consider some further chemotherapy'.

Clinician's comments: Mr Gifford has already outlived his expected prognosis. He has widespread and progressive malignant disease. He is too ill to tolerate further systemic chemotherapy but the oncologist is reluctant to say that he can 'never' have treatment again. 'Suspension' or 'postponement' of treatment is often perceived to be one way of letting people down gently, avoiding having to spell out that active treatment has stopped. However, it can lead to unrealistic expectations that more treatment will be offered in the future.[34]

During his admission Mr Gifford was assessed by the clinical oncologist and the pain specialist in order to determine whether or not palliative radiotherapy or a 'nerve block' might be helpful for his back pain. However, it was felt that his general condition was too poor to tolerate either procedure and, in any case, he had already received radiotherapy to the affected area. There were also concerns about the use of epidural injections because of a persistently low platelet count (secondary to bone marrow infiltration). After review by the palliative care team, Mr Gifford's pain was managed by increasing his morphine sulphate slow-release tablets from 60 mg to 90 mg twice per day.

The week after admission the medical team had become quite concerned about the speed of his general deterioration, and the ward sister asked the consultant to document Mr Gifford's 'resuscitation status' in the notes. Both medical and nursing staff were convinced that cardiopulmonary resuscitation (CPR) was not appropriate in this case. However, when the consultant, Dr Wigan, came to speak with Mr Gifford about resuscitation (in line with trust policy) Mr Gifford indicated that he did in fact wish to receive such treatment. Dr Wigan therefore reluctantly recorded in the notes that the patient was *for* CPR in the event of cardiorespiratory arrest. The nursing staff were very alarmed at this and did not feel that it would be ethical to attempt resuscitation in a patient with such widespread disease and in such a rapidly deteriorating condition.

*Clinician's comments: The British Medical Association, the Royal College of Nursing, and the Resuscitation Council (UK) have produced joint guidance on 'Decisions relating to cardiopulmonary resuscitation'.[35] The guidance recommends that 'where competent patients are at foreseeable risk of cardiopulmonary arrest, or have a terminal illness, there should be sensitive exploration of their wishes regarding resuscitation'. The only exception is when a patient indicates that they 'do not wish to discuss resuscitation', in which case this fact should be documented in the notes. Difficulties can arise, however, when the multi-professional team agrees that CPR would be futile but the patient nonetheless insists that he/she wishes to receive it. The BMA guidance recognises that clinicians cannot be 'required to give treatment contrary to their clinical judgment' but still recommends that patients' wishes should be respected even if 'clinical evidence suggests…that it cannot provide any overall benefit'. The dilemma that Dr Wigan and the ward nursing staff now face is a result of **following** the BMA guidance on resuscitation.[36]*

In contrast, the Association of Palliative Medicine and the National Council for Hospice and Specialist Palliative Care Services have also produced guidance on CPR in respect of patients who are terminally ill.[37] They recommend that 'there is no ethical obligation to discuss CPR with those palliative care patients for whom such treatment, following assessment, is judged to be futile'.[38]

How could Dr Wigan have handled the situation differently? The most important step is to discuss the matter within the multidisciplinary team and to come to a decision about whether CPR is clinically justifiable to offer. If there is disagreement within the team or uncertainty about the appropriateness of offering CPR, then the patient should be engaged in a genuine discussion about the benefits and burdens of the procedure and the expected outcomes. If, however, there is unanimity that CPR is not justifiable then there is no ethical obligation to discuss this with the patient because this may give the impression that the procedure is being offered (which it is not).[39] However, the clinician may feel it appropriate to inform the patient of the team's decision, to the effect that if he/she dies, the clinical team would not endeavour to restart their heart, because the chances of the procedure being successful would be extremely small, with risks outweighing the benefits.

Later that day Mr Gifford was reassessed by Dr Wigan. He had been asked by the nursing staff to speak to Mr Gifford again about the decision to *have* CPR. On this occasion Dr Wigan adopted a much more 'directive' approach to the interview and rather than asking Mr Gifford whether or not he would want to be resuscitated, he explained to Mr Gifford the reasons why the team did not feel it would be an appropriate course of action. Mr Gifford accepted that the chances of a successful outcome for CPR were negligible, and that the risks of an adverse outcome were significant. He therefore agreed that he should be *'not* for resuscitation'.

Clinician's comments: The whole process of discussing CPR status had been extremely traumatic for Mr Gifford (and his partner Sonia). They felt that a huge responsibility and burden had been placed upon their shoulders to make a 'life or death' decision about future care.[40]

The following day Dr Wigan asked Dr Taylor (the palliative care consultant) to consider transferring Mr Gifford to the local hospice for continuing care. Dr Taylor explained to Mr Gifford that the hospice would be able to offer a higher level of care for his pain control. It was explained that transfer to the hospice was not a 'one-way ticket', and that if his condition improved then he would be able to go home.

Clinician's comments: Oncologists are not the only specialists who sometimes feel the need to let patients down gently. Palliative care professionals do not always tell patients that they are being admitted to the hospice for 'terminal' or 'continuing' care. It is sometimes easier to suggest that the admission is for 'symptom control', or that if their condition improves that they will be able to go home. But just as with discussions about chemotherapy, this selective approach to truth-telling can cause problems later with unrealistic expectations.[41]

A bed became available at the hospice three days later, and Mr Gifford was transferred. On assessment at the hospice it became apparent that Mr Gifford was drowsy and confused on the current dose of morphine. He was, however, still in considerable pain, requiring breakthrough doses of oral morphine between four and five times a day. Fortunately, he found that the breakthrough doses of oral morphine were effective for the pain. However, it was noted by his partner Sonia that whenever he had a breakthrough dose he became very drowsy for the following hour. The hospice doctor felt that Mr Gifford was exhibiting some signs of opioid toxicity (sedation, confusion and myclonic jerks). However, his pain did appear to be opioid sensitive. Therefore, a decision was made to switch to an alternative opioid rather than reducing or stopping the morphine. The oral morphine was changed to a subcutaneous infusion of alfentanil (6 mg over 24 hours).

Clinician's comments: The indication for changing from morphine to an alternative opioid is a patient with opioid-sensitive pain who is experiencing intolerable side-effects with escalating doses of morphine. Alfentanil was chosen in this case because of concerns about renal impairment (alfentanil is safer to use in respect of renal failure).[42]

Initially the change of opioid resulted in an improvement in Mr Gifford's mental state. He became more lucid and less sedated. His pain, however, was not very well controlled. He continued to complain of severe pain in his thoracic spine and particularly at night became very restless because of an inability to get comfortable. He was also quite anxious about his obviously declining general state of health, and he was worrying about the effect his illness was having on his two daughters. After three days at the hospice it was noted by the staff that neither of his children had visited him. Sonia explained that the older child was busy revising for GCSE exams and that the younger child did not like to visit because of becoming upset in the hospital environment. Furthermore, it was shortly before Christmas, and Mr Gifford and his partner Sonia had arranged for their daughters to spend the holiday with grandparents in Scotland. The children had flown to Edinburgh the previous evening.

Clinician's comments: The fact that the hospice staff had not had the opportunity to speak with Mr Gifford's children was beginning to cause some alarm. The staff felt that Mr Gifford might now be dying, and they were not convinced that the children were aware of the severity of his condition.

Initially, Mr Gifford was reluctant to agree to an increase in his regular analgesia because he wished 'to keep a clear head'. However, he was requiring frequent breakthrough doses of alfentanil (sometimes as often as eight times a day). Over the next few days his pain escalated further, and with agreement from Mr Gifford, the pump rate was increased first to 12 mg and then to 20 mg of alfentanil per 24 hours. A decision was also taken to add in a small amount of midazolam (a sedative) in order to relax the patient and reduce some of his agitation. Sonia was becoming increasingly anxious and distressed at seeing her partner in frequent pain.

Clinician's comments: Although Mr Gifford had widespread disease he did not feel 'ready to die yet'. He did not wish to be confused or sedated, but neither did he wish to be in pain.[43]

At the higher dose of alfentanil and with the concomitant use of midazolam, Mr Gifford eventually became peaceful. Unfortunately the escalating doses of opiates had resulted in him becoming very sedated and unable to communicate with Sonia. At this point it became readily apparent that Mr Gifford was in the terminal phase of his illness. Sonia decided to call her parents in Scotland and to summon the girls back to the hospice so that they could be with their father at the end. By the time that the girls arrived at the hospice their father was comfortable but sedated. Sonia became extremely concerned that the girls had not had a chance to say goodbye and speak to their father properly. Furthermore, she was feeling guilty that she had agreed to them going away to Scotland.

Clinician's comments: Sonia had been trying to 'protect' her children from the reality of their father's condition. But now that he is clearly dying it has become apparent that the truth can no longer be concealed from them.[44] She is feeling guilty that she deprived the children of the opportunity to speak to their father when he was more lucid. In fact, it is highly likely that the children had a good insight into how ill their father was, but they were content to participate in the charade that Sonia played for their benefit.[45]

Sonia asked to speak to the palliative care consultant. She was concerned that her partner was now being given too much alfentanil and that this was keeping him sedated when, if he had the choice, he might have preferred to be more awake so that he could speak to his daughters. Sonia was also concerned that the large doses of alfentanil might be hastening his death.[46]

Clinician's comments: Mr Gifford is clearly now much more comfortable than he has been for several weeks – unfortunately he is also quite heavily sedated. The sedation is an unintended consequence of the analgesia. Every effort had been made to control his pain without causing undue sedation (including a switch from morphine to alfentanil), but unfortunately it had not been possible to achieve both goals. Mr Gifford was never directly asked whether or not he wished to be sedated but it was noted that during the preceding few weeks he had been asking for frequent 'breakthrough' doses of analgesia regardless of how drowsy he was feeling. This was taken to indicate that analgesia was a higher priority than maintaining a clearer level of consciousness.

Alfentanil per se would be unlikely to hasten Mr Gifford's death. The dose had been titrated against his pain and was not causing respiratory depression. His advanced and rapidly progressive disease meant that his life expectancy at this stage was only likely to be a few days at best. If Mr Gifford were not to die from his underlying disease within a few days, and were he not to be given artificial hydration, then alfentanil might indirectly hasten his death by causing dehydration. However, this could be prevented by the provision of subcutaneous fluids, even though alfentanil may also indirectly hasten his death by predisposing him to developing a respiratory tract infection.

The palliative care consultant discussed the issues with Sonia and suggested that they could try reducing the dose of midazolam (the sedative) in an effort to improve his conscious level. However, the consultant explained that she felt it was unlikely that this would result in any great improvement in mental awareness. The other possibility that was discussed was to reduce the alfentanil dosage, but the palliative care consultant was reluctant to do this because the last 24 hours had been the first time that Mr Gifford had looked comfortable since his admission to the hospice 10 days previously.

Clinician's comments: The clinician's primary duty is to care for the patient, and for this reason the palliative care consultant was reluctant to agree to any alteration in the alfentanil dosage. However, he was sympathetic to Sonia's concerns that Mr Gifford might not wish to be quite so sedated, and might wish to have the opportunity to speak with his family again. For this reason the palliative care consultant suggested a small reduction in the midazolam dosage (although this did have a potential problem of causing an exacerbation of Mr Gifford's agitation).

Matters were further complicated when Mr Gifford's parents arrived from Scotland. They did not wish the midazolam or alfentanil doses to be reduced because they had seen Guy suffering from severe pain for several weeks prior to admission to the hospice. They did not feel that anything valuable would be gained by reducing the level of sedation, and felt that this was only likely to cause unnecessary distress. After discussion within the family and with the medical and nursing staff, a decision was taken not to alter the dosage of any of the drugs. Mr Gifford died peacefully the following morning with his family at his bedside.[47]

Case history 5: Farida Fatah

Abstract
Mrs Fatah is a 75-year-old woman with widespread lung cancer. She lives in Dubai and has come over to the UK for private treatment. She speaks no English and her family translate on her behalf. The family is reluctant to give Mrs Fatah accurate information about her condition and does not allow independent translators to intervene. It is not clear that Mrs Fatah is able to give informed consent to her medical treatment.

Case history 5
Mrs Fatah was a 75-year-old woman who lived in Dubai and spoke no English. She arrived in the UK with her two sons who were able to translate for her. She was seen as a private patient by an orthopaedic surgeon for the investigation and management of a painful left shoulder. Investigations soon revealed widespread cancer affecting her bones, and further investigations revealed that she had a stage IV (inoperable) non-small cell cancer affecting the right lung. The disease was locally extensive and was causing erosion of the anterior left ribs. She was seen by Dr Marshall (a clinical oncologist), who felt that some palliative radiotherapy may help with the management of her pain and dyspnoea. During all of the consultations Mrs Fatah was seen with her two sons, who acted as translators.

Clinician's comments: Mrs Fatah's disease is incurable and she has a short-term prognosis. She has been seen by several doctors (and nurses) and all members of staff have used her sons as translators. Although this is often the most convenient method of communication with non-English speakers, it can lead to ethical and practical problems.[48]

Although full and frank disclosure took place with Mrs Fatah's sons, it soon became clear that they were unwilling to translate all relevant information and communicate it to their mother. They explained that they did not feel that it was 'culturally appropriate' for their mother to know the full extent of her illness.[49]

Clinician's comments: Although Mrs Fatah had already undergone numerous tests and investigations, her lack of understanding about her illness only became apparent when her written consent was required for a specific medical procedure.

The clinical oncologist asked Mrs Fatah whether she would like a professional translator rather than one of her sons to act as a translator for her, but she indicated that she preferred to have her family involved. Her sons became quite angry that Dr Marshall had suggested involving someone 'independent', and they felt that he did not trust them to translate honestly. They admitted that they did not translate everything exactly but explained that this was because they knew that their mother did not wish to know the details, and that she had entrusted her sons to make appropriate decisions on behalf.[50]

Clinician's comments: Dr Marshall's effort to challenge Mrs Fatah's sons had resulted in a breakdown of trust between the family and the medical staff. As far as Dr Marshall could tell the sons had translated accurately his offer of an 'independent translator' and Mrs Fatah had genuinely rejected the offer. However, it was difficult to be absolutely certain and Dr Marshall did not feel that further confrontation (for example, by arranging an independent translator, despite the sons' stated wishes) would be helpful. To a large extent these problems could have been avoided if an independent translator had been used at the outset; Mrs Fatah could then have been seen alone. However, practical constraints usually mean that family members are used instead.

The following day, Dr Marshall explained to Mrs Fatah (with translation by one of her sons) the need for radiotherapy in order to treat her underlying cancer. The son translated this by explaining that 'x-ray treatment' was needed for her 'chest pain'. No explanation was made relating to the presence or otherwise of cancer.[51]

Clinician's comments: This would clearly not be a 'fully informed' consent. Nonetheless, Mrs Fatah understood the nature of the treatment that she was agreeing to and the expected side-effects. She understood the purpose of the treatment (to palliate the pain in her chest) even if she did not explicitly understand the underlying diagnosis. Dr Marshall reasoned that Mrs Fatah knew enough to consent to the treatment, and in all likelihood she understood that she had cancer.

Following this discussion Mrs Fatah consented to the radiotherapy. However, despite starting treatment, she died suddenly one week later from a probable pulmonary embolus (clot on the lung).

Case history 6: Barbara Bowen

Abstract
Mrs Bowen is an 80-year-old lady with advanced colon cancer. Her condition deteriorates and she starts to die. However, her terminal phase is longer than anticipated and this becomes a source of conflict between clinical staff and Mrs Bowen's family.

Case history 6
Mrs Bowen was an 80-year-old retired shopkeeper. She suffered from advanced metastatic colon cancer. She had been diagnosed five years previously and been treated with surgery, radiotherapy and more recently with palliative chemotherapy. She now had progressive disease and had been admitted to hospital for symptom control because of uncontrolled pain.

On examination she was a frail lady with a mini mental test score of 20 out of 20. She was in obvious discomfort at rest. She had bony tenderness in the left hip joint and neuropathic (nerve) pain down the left leg. Routine biochemistry and haematology on admission were unremarkable. Investigations revealed widespread bony deposits with a 'hot spot' on the bone scan corresponding to the painful area in her left sacroiliac joint.

Clinician's comments: Mrs Bowen had advanced, progressive and incurable cancer. Her investigations revealed that her pain was due to the cancer spreading to her bones. She was not confused.[52]

Plans were made to treat Mrs Bowen with palliative radiotherapy to the painful bony lesion. In the meantime she was started on four-hourly morphine in combination with non-steroidal anti-inflammatory drugs and antidepressants (for the nerve pain).

Clinician's comments: This is standard therapy for this type of pain.

Two weeks after admission, while still waiting for radiotherapy, Mrs Bowen's condition suddenly deteriorated. Blood tests revealed that she had developed acute renal failure. An ultrasound scan revealed that this was secondary to bilateral hydronephrosis (obstruction of the kidneys due to cancer in the pelvis). She was reviewed by the urology team, who concluded that her general condition rendered her too frail for any surgical intervention.

Clinician's comments: In fitter patients the obstruction could be relieved by inserting drainage tubes directly into the kidney. However, in this case the urologists felt that Mrs Bowen was too frail to be able to tolerate the procedure. There was also a question as to whether this type of treatment would have been in her best interests. Just because ureteric obstruction can be relatively easily reversed does not mean that it is always appropriate to do so. Treating the obstruction may result in a brief prolongation of life but in the long run may lead to more suffering and debility. Everybody has to die of 'something' and there is sometimes a tendency in medical care to only allow patients to die when they are somehow in a state of perfect health...[53]

Mrs Bowen accepted that her condition was terminal and was relieved that further active intervention was not planned. She was, however, quite tearful and distressed about her situation. She requested that she be given some sedation to ease her agitation. This was discussed with both Mrs Bowen and her family, and a syringe driver was started containing midazolam 15 mg (a sedative with anxiety-relieving effects) and diamorphine 15 mg (a pain killer) administered subcutaneously by syringe driver over 24 hours.

Clinician's comments: It is important that the clinician checks that Mrs Bowen is still competent to make these kinds of decision about her medical care. She was not confused on admission, and she was competent to make decisions at that time. The doctor ensured that this was still the case when reassessing the situation on this occasion. It was explained that this treatment would 'relax' her and keep her comfortable although it would result in increased drowsiness.

After 24 hours Mrs Bowen's condition deteriorated and she became semi-conscious. Her family kept a bedside vigil for 48 hours. During this time Mrs Bowen occasionally showed signs that she was still able to hear what people were saying to her but she was unable or unwilling to respond to them.[54]

Clinician's comments: The 'death bed vigil' can be an exhausting ordeal for family members and staff. Relatives and carers often wish to be with their loved ones at the moment of death. For this reason staff sometimes call relatives in the middle of the night if they suspect that a patient is imminently dying. However, clinical staff are not always very accurate at judging when death is imminent, and occasionally family and friends can be kept in a state of constant alert for many days. After a while, carers become anxious at leaving the bedside for even a moment (to wash, visit the bathroom or sleep) in case they are not present at the moment of death.

However, after 48 hours Mrs Bowen's condition if anything seemed to be improving. She was awake for more of the day than she was asleep. She was occasionally speaking coherently, although at other times her speech appeared to consist of nonsense phrases. This change in Mrs Bowen's condition caused some consternation and distress to both her family and to the medical and nursing staff on the ward. The supposition had been that Mrs Bowen was imminently dying and this change in her condition was unsettling for all concerned.

The palliative care team was called to see Mrs Bowen. She indicated to them that she was not in pain and was comfortable. However, when further questions were asked of her, she was unable to give a coherent answer.[55] On examination there were some signs of mild dehydration although she was still passing some urine via her catheter. A discussion was then undertaken with members of Mrs Bowen's family, who were quite distressed at her apparent recovery. They felt that she had said her goodbyes and that she was ready to die. They reported that she had told them that she did not 'wish to linger', and they were sure that she would not have wanted to be maintained in her current condition. There was some disagreement among the family members about the correct way to proceed. Some wished for her sedation to be increased, others felt that it should be reduced. Furthermore there was disagreement about whether or not it was appropriate to provide artificial fluids for Mrs Bowen.[56]

Clinician's comments: Mrs Bowen's illness did not follow the path predicted by the doctors and anticipated by the relatives. The palliative care team had to balance a number of conflicting demands in order adequately to address the clinical situation. The team's first priority had to be towards the patient – but what did she want? To all intents and purposes she was comfortable and not agitated. However, her family felt that 'if she could see herself now' she would prefer to be more deeply sedated (or indeed that she would prefer to be dead). It was also apparent that the family was exhausted by the longer than expected terminal phase of Mrs Bowen's illness and was keen for it 'all to be over'. The staff were finding it emotionally draining to look after a patient who seemed to be lingering in the hinterland between death and life, but the palliative care team was conscious of not wishing to hasten Mrs Bowen's death ('because it would be easier all round'), even though they did not wish unnecessarily to prolong her dying.[57]

After considering all of the factors the palliative care team started Mrs Bowen on subcutaneous fluids (1 litre of normal saline over 24 hours) and her sedation was left unaltered. Over the next 48 hours her condition remained essentially unchanged. She was still opening her eyes and occasionally communicating verbally and did not appear to be in any distress. She was unable to take any fluid orally. After 72 hours her condition deteriorated once again and she became unconscious. She remained in this condition for a further 72 hours before dying peacefully with her family at her bedside.

Clinician's comments: Mrs Bowen ended up requiring sedation for nine days prior to death. Her family was at her bedside for this entire period. Although her prolonged dying phase was originally a source of concern and distress to the family, ultimately family members became reconciled to 'letting nature take her course in her own time'. They felt that Mrs Bowen's dying reflected her manner of living ('no one was going to tell her how to do it') and the family was glad that her death had not been hastened.[58]

Notes to Part Two

[1] It is important for the clinical team to be able to establish an accurate diagnosis; it is also important for the patient to know what is going on and what each procedure entails in terms of associated risk. Separate consent would normally be required for each different test.

[2] No matter how well procedures are followed in terms of formal consent, ultimately it is a question of how well it is performed by the responsible clinician that determines whether or not it achieves its objective in terms of providing patient-centred care and enabling a properly informed choice. The difficulty here is that potentially these two objectives could be in conflict, one with the other.

[3] This was the right path to follow, even though Mrs Adair's instincts suggested otherwise. She was not to blame in any way, as she was only looking out for her husband's best interests. Such a situation needed to be handled with firmness and sensitivity, as appeared to be the case here. Mr Adair had to be given the chance to make his own choices; as things turned out, events did lead to a temporary loss of capacity.

[4] This was a helpful intervention to make, counterbalancing increasing medicalisation of the patient's care.

[5] A case of good open communication and teamwork.

[6] Medical staff are not always willing to engage in this type of discussion, and the palliative care team did well to raise these issues, even though in this case the patient was not especially interested. In other cases, lack of responsiveness to such issues by a medical team could cause real distress.

[7] This case is not atypical in that the patient's condition deteriorated after a previous instruction had not been accurately followed; clinical error often results from poor communication. The intervention in this case did affect how the case was managed at that point, but it did not amount to any sort of clinical negligence, and ultimately made no difference to later disease progression.

[8] This case illustrates well some of the problems discussed in Chapters 4 and 6.

[9] There is no suggestion here that the doctrine of double effect be brought into play and in this instance it would be unnecessary and inappropriate.

[10] The patient did not succeed in having his final wish to be allowed to die in the surroundings of his own home. This was in a sense unfortunate but, given the necessary medicalisation of his care and rapid deterioration of the patient in the final phase, was really unavoidable. It is difficult for anyone to try and claim it as a 'right' to be allowed to die at home. Much depends on the circumstances of each case, such as the degree of medical management needed and the family situation. While in this case the patient's wife may have been happy for her husband to be allowed home, it would have been the likely cause of considerable stress to her as the primary carer, as well as possibly impacting on the wider family. It is better, therefore, to avoid generalisable claims in this regard.

[11] At this point in the narrative it is the clinical aspects of the case that are dominant. The more ethical dimensions become apparent later on.

[12] This fact is crucial, because if there are no valid treatment options that can address the underlying condition, then everything centres on how the case is managed. This is different from situations where there are various treatment options available, and where risks and benefits can be weighed carefully, one against another. In terminal cases such as this, choices have to be made within a narrow framework of options, and may relate simply to which treatment is 'least bad' or has the fewest side-effects (i.e. relative to the benefits of palliation).

[13] The decision to stop the particular medicat   ion was taken by the hospital team before Mr Deakin was referred for palliative care. It would imply that the oncology team believed that Karen had a *right* to influence the decision, which was not in fact the case.

[14] Karen is trying to overstep the line here and needs to stand back. She has no authority to make decisions, and while she can reasonably contribute to discussions about her father's care, she has no authority to act as his proxy decision-maker.

[15] *See* Chapter 3.

[16] Karen perhaps needs support to help her deal with the trauma surrounding her father's illness; her interventions are not helpful either to the clinical team or necessarily to her father. Patients in a weakened condition can benefit greatly from having someone to advocate on their behalf and interact with the clinical team, but there are good and bad ways of doing this.

[17] *See* Chapter 6.

[18] In that instance the patient's wishes would be binding on the clinical team.

[19] Here, however, things are different and the team would have to decide whether or not Mr Deakin would have wanted the additional medication had he been competent to decide for himself. In addition, the team would have to ask themselves if potential benefits of medicating outweighed the perceived risks. In the case of opiate analgesics, this can mean life being shortened to some extent. Provided there is no intention to hasten death then such prescribing is perfectly acceptable and falls under the heading of double effect (i.e. where a patient suffers unintentional but foreseeable harm (including death) without any suspicion of blame falling on the clinician). There is nothing to suggest that Mr Deakin was losing capacity early in the narrative, but once he was taking diazepam (and subsequently diamorphine), the matter became less clear. Patients can lose capacity as a direct result of the medication they are taking, and while theoretically this can be controlled, in practical terms it is difficult to stop giving medication just in order to ask the patient 'Do you consent to us giving you x, y or z?', and in any case, confusion may be attributable to the underlying medical condition, not the treatment itself.

In non-terminal cases where, for instance, major surgery is planned, then a surgical team has no authority to act if there is any possibility that a patient can be brought round to the point at which it became possible for the team to explain the risks and benefits, and thus for the patient to make a reasonably informed decision. The clinical threshold for capacity is relatively low, so this may not present a major difficulty. But how meaningful a consent is, say, in the intensive care setting where a patient is unstable or in a life-threatening situation is open to some doubt. Consent may be legally valid without it necessarily conforming to the highest ethical standards. Note the earlier comment about practical ethics being a 'messy business'. The 'best interests argument' is the best there is (under current English law) and in theory ought to be sufficient to protect patients from unjustified treatment with no likely benefit and high risk.

[20] This was probably more of an emotional than a reasoned response, with the daughter being unwilling to accept the inevitable.

[21] Such treatment would not be considered radical on a 54-year-old patient, but even a *fit* 94-year-old would be hard pressed to withstand this amount of surgical intervention.

[22] Not all forms of discrimination are wrong *per se*. To discriminate simply means to allow one's judgment to be influenced by external factors, in particular, those which cannot be controlled. It is *unfair* discrimination that is unethical, and in most medical decisions, age is a variable that cannot be changed, but which nonetheless needs to be taken into consideration. In this case it was an entirely reasonable thing to factor into discussions about the treatment plan.

[23] This is a classic case of 'success' being measured (in medical terms) as 'a life saved', i.e. not one well lived. A more successful outcome might be one that does not subject a patient to aggressive intervention for such an uncertain benefit. Extending life is not an unconditional benefit and needs to be qualified by other considerations relating to quality of life and, where possible, the express wishes of the patient.

24 Given the circumstances, the term 'cure' may not be an appropriate concept about which to be thinking.

25 Unfortunately, 'best interests' can be used to justify what a clinician wants, and not what the patient may or may not have wanted.

26 This is what is implied by saying the case has its own momentum. The son was now convinced of the wisdom of carrying out the operations. Although the first round of surgery resulted in nothing untoward, it had not done anything directly to address the main condition. Mr Evans (Snr.) now faced the prospect of a second operation, this time to his primary tumour. At this stage it is possibly too late to stand back and take an objective view about the whole process of managing this particular patient.

27 If the patient still has legal capacity he is fully within his rights in refusing further treatment, even though his life depends on it. There is adequate legal precedent for this to be accepted as fact. However, matters become a little murky when questions are raised about the patient's capacity to decide, and it is not unlikely that, given what this patient has recently been through, his relative incapacity is a direct result of medical intervention. This leaves him somewhat at the mercy of the clinical team to decide what is 'in his best interests'. Palliative care is almost certainly the best option for him now, and in fact, may well have been for quite some time.

28 i.e. he is able to satisfy the normal criteria for making a capacitous decision.

29 In the circumstances this was a good way to proceed.

30 This document can be downloaded from the UK Department of Health website: www.dh.gov.uk/PublicationsAndStatistics/Publications/PublicationsPolicyAndGuidance/PublicationsPolicyAndGuidanceArticle/fs/en?CONTENT_ID=4006757&chk=snmdw8.

31 This is a slightly strange way of speaking, and it is not clear what is behind the intention to try to 'make' the patient get better other than to try and justify further intervention.

32 Over-riding a patient's clearly articulated wishes and, contrary to those wishes, continuing with active treatment is a form of assault unless it is considered that the patient's wishes are suicidal. In this case Mr Evans was not requesting that treatment should be stopped so as to bring about his own death (he would after all have been only too happy to make a swift recovery from surgery) – instead it was because he found the treatment unduly onerous. The surgical and palliative care teams did not feel that Mr Evans' request was suicidal in nature.

33 Consent is an ongoing process rather than a single act. Although Mr Evans had previously agreed to aggressive treatment he is not bound by his previous decisions. It may seem 'illogical' to agree to invasive surgery and then to refuse even antibiotics, but Mr Evans' circumstances have changed considerably, and he is at liberty to decide how active he wishes his ongoing management to be. To ignore clearly stated, competently formed wishes may expose clinical staff and the hospital to legal suit for unauthorised clinical intervention.

34 There are issues here about truth-telling and when it is acceptable to withhold information in a patient's best interests. While there may not be a clear line that can be drawn here, the tendency is increasingly towards disclosure. This is appropriate because it empowers the patient to make decisions for themselves when there are decisions to be made. In situations where there is no actual decision to make, proper disclosure allows patients to adjust to their new circumstances, and perhaps to make arrangements to see their family one last time. Not all patients want this kind of information, however, and to give too much information or at the wrong time can cause harm. While it is a judgment call deciding what information to disclose and what to withhold, care has to be taken not to be paternalistic in withholding information. Current consent law requires that there has to be adequate justification in support of *non*-disclosure (*see* Chapter 4).

35 British Medical Association *et al.* (2001).

36 For a full discussion of the BMA position, see British Medical Association (2003: Chapter 10). *See also* Chapter 4.

37 This information can be viewed via the Council's website: www.hospice-spc-council.org.uk.

38 This situation is not atypical. It is quite common for different sets of guidelines to offer differing advice on how to respond in a given situation. Guidelines issued by various bodies can contain contradictory or inconsistent advice. This situation arises for a number of reasons. Among them are policy confusion, a failure to implement practice guidance, a lack of agreement amongst practising professionals, and sometimes lack of clarity in the law. Common law judgments have to be applied with discretion relative to the merits of an individual case, and *statute* law does not often apply in relation to routine clinical practice. While it is generally left to qualified professionals to determine what is considered best practice, the situation is changing as more and more guidelines are being produced.

39 Actions may be in accord with a consensus view of how a given situation should be handled, but judgment still has to be exercised in determining how, if or when to follow guidance. Ethically speaking, it would be inappropriate to attempt CPR at this stage, and were it not for the fact that the patient had requested it in advance, resuscitation (determined by balance of harms and general clinical futility) could have amounted to battery.

40 Reference has already been made to the possibility of harm being done by providing too much information or at the wrong time; here it is the burden of emotional harm that is the issue. It can be a difficult call deciding whether to accept a patient's reluctance to address the issues at hand and respect an autonomous choice *not* to be fully informed, or to press ahead and alert the patient (and his/her family) to present realities, and so to the possibility of imminent death. Consent is invalid if improperly informed, so if a patient refuses to discuss serious issues, then one course of action would be to ask the patient to delegate authority back to the clinician to do what s/he thinks best. However, best practice indicates that patients, when competent, should be fully involved in decisions about their care, so 'upwards' delegation is not a preferred course of action.

41 Truth-telling is almost always the best option.

42 This decision is based on clinical criteria, the only ethical implication being that capacity is likely to be impaired by administration of high levels of morphine. But high levels of pain also impair judgment, making it all the more important to attend to the question of pain control (*see* Chapter 6).

43 It is not always easy to achieve a balance, and in this the patient is unclear as to which matters most – pain control or trying to keep a clear mind (*see* Chapter 6). The team is right to be worried about the children, because it may soon be too late to bring them in.

44 For practical advice on how to tell children about a parent's diagnosis see CancerLink (2001).

45 The mother is acting in what she perceives as the children's best interests, even though the reality may well be different.

46 *See* Chapters 4 and 6 on the doctrine of double effect.

47 The final outcome was never really in doubt. While this case would not have been easy to manage, there was less open conflict than in other cases. It could be argued that overall this was a 'good result' in that the patient died (from his underlying condition) in relative comfort, and in the company of his immediate family.

48 The situation described is not uncommon, and it can be expected that patients will need treatment in situations where there is no common language for communication. For practical reasons professional translators are not always available, so it often falls

to relatives attending to act as intermediaries between doctor and patient. If the patient herself is in agreement with these arrangements then ethically speaking it need not be problematic. Some hospitals use volunteers to act as translators, but general hospitals, especially in areas of high ethnic diversity, can be presented with any number of languages needing translation, quite apart from temporary situations arising from holiday or business travel, or travel for the sake of medical treatment itself, as in the present case.

49 Deliberate withholding of information from a patient is not appropriate according to standards of practice widely employed in the West. However, it is entirely appropriate for relatives to demonstrate social and cultural respect for a sick member of their family. To do otherwise could easily destroy the trust that exists between family members. It would also be disrespectful towards cultural values that differed from one's own. The culture of informed consent is essentially based on a Western ethic, and respect for patient autonomy cannot be assumed to have equal moral status in different cultures.

50 Patients do not have to be told all there is to know about their condition if they do not want to hear. It is good practice to try to persuade patients to listen and take part in discussions about their care, but they cannot be forced to do so. It is more difficult where an intermediary is relied upon to act as a faithful translator. However, family members in this case were merely acting as health proxies for their mother. She had legal capacity but was unable to exercise that capacity because of language barriers, and exercising 'deferred autonomy' via the sons was probably the best available option. A question remains, though, of whose culture should prevail and in which circumstance. Mrs Fatah and her sons are acting respectfully towards their own cultural traditions, but the clinical team is bound by their own local ethical and legal codes, which cannot be ignored. Trust in family relationships is equally as important in this situation as the trust between patient and doctor, even if the former is not bound by explicit ethical codes.

51 The sons were not ethically 'out of order' even if they did not do exactly as they were asked by the clinical oncologist. If the situation were reversed, say with the consultant ill in a hospital in Dubai while attending a conference, he could not expect English laws and customs to be followed at that hospital, and he might need a translator himself. He might also want full and frank disclosure about his medical condition and may not be pleased to receive a paternalistic response from his doctor. He may probably benefit himself from having someone to hand to act as health proxy, but his rights as a patient would ultimately be bound by prevailing *local* laws and customs.

52 So far, the case is straightforward and the patient clearly has legal capacity.

53 This may sound odd but there is some truth to it, and the point has already been made that death is often viewed as a kind of failure.

54 It is at this stage that capacity is impaired to the point where the patient is effectively unable to exercise her autonomy. While capacity may be lacking, the team at this stage has some knowledge of the patient and her wishes. The family is also in attendance, and so her incapacity is not unduly problematic in terms of trying to establish her wishes.

55 Clearly her capacity is considerably impaired by this point, but that does not mean that it is inappropriate to try to involve her in decisions about her care, and her capacity level may well continue to fluctuate.

56 From a legal point of view, the supply of artificial hydration has some significance. To withdraw it would almost certainly hasten death, and failure to provide it would probably be thought cruel and likely to cause increased suffering (*see* Chapter 6).

57 There is no suggestion here that practical measures were ever being considered to deliberately hasten her death.

58 It would be interesting to reconsider this case but with the addition of an advance statement. Had the patient written a living will it could have influenced the practical course of events, possibly complicating the issue without there being any overall benefit. It must not be assumed that advance statements are automatically 'a good thing' or, for that matter, something best avoided.

References and further reading

References

Alderson P and Goodey C (1998) Theories of consent. *BMJ*. **317**: 1313–15.

Beauchamp TL and Childress JF (1994) *Biomedical Ethics* (4e). Oxford University Press, Oxford.

Beel A, McClement SE and Harlos M (2002) Palliative sedation therapy: a review of definitions and usage. *Internat J Pall Nurs*. **8**(4): 190–99.

Bentham J (1968) *The Collected Works of Jeremy Bentham*. Athlone Press, London.

Billings JA and Block SD (1996) Slow euthanasia. *J Pall Care*. **12**(4): 21–30.

Bratjman S (2003) The impact on the family of terminal restlessness and its management. *Pall Med*. **17**(5): 454–60.

Bridson J, Hammond C, Leach A *et al.* (2003) Making consent patient centred. *BMJ*. **327**: 1159–61.

Bristol Royal Infirmary Inquiry (2001) *Learning from Bristol: the report of the public enquiry into children's heart surgery at the Bristol Royal Infirmary 1984 –1995*. www.bristol-inquiry.org.uk/final report.

British Medical Association (2003) *Medical Ethics Today* (2e). BMA, London.

British Medical Association, Resuscitation Council (UK) and Royal College of Nursing (2001) Decisions Relating to Cardiopulmonary Resuscitation (a joint statement). *J Med Eth*. **27**: 312–18.

CancerLink (2001) *Talking to Children When an Adult has Cancer*. CancerLink, London.

Chan KS, Sham MMK, Tse DMW *et al.* (2004) Palliative medicine in malignant respiratory diseases. In: D Doyle, G Hanks, N Cherny *et al.* (eds) *Oxford Textbook of Palliative Medicine* (3e). Oxford University Press, Oxford.

Chater S, Viola R, Paterson J *et al.* (1998) Sedation for intractable distress in the dying: a survey of experts. *Pall Med*. **12**: 255–69.

Cherny NI and Portenoy RK (1994) Sedation in the management of refractory symptoms: guidelines for evaluation and treatment. *J Pall Care*. **10**(2): 31–8.

Chiu TY, Hu WY, Lue BH *et al.* (2001) Sedation for refractory symptoms of terminal cancer patients in Taiwan. *J Pain Symp Manage*.**21**: 467–72.

Chochinov HM *et al.* (1995) Desire for death in the terminally ill. *Am J Psych*. **152**: 1185–91.

Coleman J and Shapiro S (eds) (2004) *The Oxford Handbook of Jurisprudence and Philosophy of Law*. Oxford University Press, Oxford.

Coleman JL (2001) *The Practice of Principle*. Oxford University Press, Oxford.

Corner J (1997) More openness needed in palliative care. *BMJ*. **315**: 242.

Crisp R (ed.) (1998) *Utilitarianism (Oxford Philosophical Texts)*. Oxford University Press, Oxford.

Doyle D, Hanks GW and MacDonald N (eds) (1998) *Oxford Textbook of Palliative Medicine* (2e). Oxford University Press, Oxford.

Dworkin R (1986) *Law's Empire*. Harvard University Press, Cambridge, Mass.

Dworkin R (2000) *Sovereign Virtue*. Harvard University Press, Cambridge, Mass.

Dyer O (2004) Man wins battle to keep receiving life support. *BMJ*. **329**: 309.

Ellershaw JE and Ward C (2003) Care of the dying patient: the last hours or days of life. *BMJ*. **326**: 30–4.

Fainsinger RL, de Moissac D, Mancini I *et al.* (2000a) Sedation for delirium and other symptoms in terminally ill patients in Edmonton. *J Pall Care* **16**(2): 5–10.

Fainsinger R, Waller A, Bercovici M *et al.* (2000b) A multicentre international study of sedation for uncontrolled symptoms in terminally ill patients. *Pall Med*. **14**: 257–65.

Fainsinger RL, Nunez-Olarte JM and Demoissac DM (2003) The cultural differences in perceived value of disclosure and cognition: Spain and Canada. *J Pall Care*. **19**(1): 43–8.

General Medical Council (1998) *Seeking Patients' Consent: the ethical considerations*. GMC, London.

General Medical Council (2002) *Withholding and Withdrawing Life-prolonging Treatments: good practice in decision-making*. GMC, London.

Hart HLA (1964) *The Concept of Law*. Oxford University Press, Oxford.

Hart HLA (2001) *Essays on Bentham: jurisprudence and political theory*. Oxford University Press, Oxford.

Hattab AS (2004) Current trends in teaching ethics of healthcare practices. *Developing World Bioethics*. **4**(2): 160–72.

Hawryluck LA, Harvey WRC, Lemieux-Charles L *et al.* (2002) Consensus guidelines on analgesia and sedation in dying intensive care unit patients. *BMC Med Eth*. **3**: 3. www.biomedcentral.com/1472-6939/3/3.

Horton R (2001) The real lessons from Harold Frederick Shipman. *Lancet*. **357**: 82–3.

Keown J (2002) *Euthanasia, Ethics and Public Policy*. Cambridge University Press, Cambridge.

Ladd J (trans.) (1999) Immanuel Kant, metaphysics of morals. In: *Metaphysical Elements of Justice* (2e). Hackett, London.

Locke J (1979) *John Locke: an essay concerning human understanding* (ed. PH Nidditch). Oxford University Press, Oxford.

Macklin R (2003) Dignity is a useless concept. *BMJ*. **327**: 1419–20.

Marks P (2003) The evolution of the doctrine of consent. *Clin Med J Roy Coll Physicians*. **3**: 45–7.

Mayberry MK and Mayberry JF (2002) Consent with understanding: a movement towards informed decisions. *Clin Med J Roy Coll Physicians*. **2**: 523–6.

McGee G (ed.) (2003) *Pragmatic Bioethics* (2e). Massachusetts Institute of Technology Press, Massachusetts.

McIver B, Walsh D and Nelson K (1994) The use of chlorpromazine for symptom control in dying cancer patients. *J Pain Symp Manage*. **9**: 341–5.

Meystre CJN, Burley NMJ and Ahmedzai S (1997) What investigations and procedures do patients in hospices want? Interview-based study of patients and their nurses. *BMJ*. **315**: 1202–3.

Mills JS (1984) *Utilitarianism* (ed. G Sher). Hackett, London.

Morgan D (1997) *Readings in Thanatology*. Baywood Publishing Company, New York.

Morita T, Inoue S and Chihara S (1996) Sedation for symptom control in Japan: the importance of intermittent use and communication with family members. *J Pain Symp Manage*. **12**: 32–8.

Morita T, Tsunoda J, Inoue S *et al.* (1999) Do hospice clinicians sedate patients intending to hasten death? *J Pall Care.* **15**(3): 20–3.

Morita T, Tsuneto S and Shima Y (2002) Definition of sedation for symptom relief: a systematic literature review and a proposal of operational criteria. *J Pain Symp Manage.* **24**(4): 447–53.

Morita T, Hirai K, Akechi T *et al.* (2003) Similarity and difference among standard medical care, palliative sedation therapy and euthanasia: a multidimensional scaling analysis on physicians and the general population's opinions. *J Pain Symp Manage.* **25**: 357–62.

Muller-Busch HC, Andres I and Jehser T (2003) Sedation in palliative care: a critical analysis of 7 years experience. *BMC Pall Care.* **2**: 2. www.biomed-central.com/1472-684X/2/2.

Murtagh F and Thorns A (2003) *The evaluation of using an ethics history with hospice in-patients.* Poster presentation. EAPC Conference, The Hague.

National Institute for Clinical Excellence (2004) *Supportive and Palliative Care Cancer Service Guidance.* http://www.nice.org.uk/page.aspx?o=110005.

Parekh B (2004) How Universal are Human Rights? Oxford Amnesty Lecture. *Times Higher Education Supplement*, February 6.

Posner R (2002) *Problematics of Moral and Legal Theory.* Belknap Press, Harvard, Mass.

Quill TE and Byock IR (2000) Responding to intractable terminal suffering: the role of terminal sedation and voluntary refusal of food and fluids. *Ann Intern Med.* **132**: 402–14.

Quill TE, Lo B and Brock DW (1997) Palliative options of last resort: a comparison of voluntary stopping eating and drinking, terminal sedation, physician assisted suicide and voluntary active euthanasia. *JAMA.* **278**(23): 2099–104.

Randall F and Downie R (2004) Truth-telling and consent. In: D Doyle, G Hanks, N Cherny *et al.* (eds) *Oxford Textbook of Palliative Medicine* (3e). Oxford University Press, Oxford.

Rawls J (2001) *Theory of Justice* (revised edn). Harvard University Press, Harvard, Mass.

Rawls J, Fried C and Sen A (1987) *Liberty, Equality and Law: selected Tanner lectures on moral philosophy.* University of Utah Press, Utah.

Ross D (2002) Game theory. In: E N Zalta (ed.) *The Stanford (online) Encyclopedia of Philosophy* (spring edition). http://plato.stanford.edu/archives/spr2002/entries/game-theory/.

Rowe M (2002a) *The Book of Jesse.* The Francis Press, Washington DC.

Rowe M (2002b) The rest is silence. *Health Affairs.* **21**(4): 232–6.

Russell B (1938) *Principles of Mathematics.* Norton & Company, New York. First published 1903.

Sales JP (2001) Sedation and terminal care. *Eur J Pall Care.* **8**: 97–100.

Sayers GM *et al.* (2001) The value of taking an 'ethics history'. *J Med Eth.* **27**: 114–17.

Shapiro S (2002) Law, plans, and practical reason. *Legal Theory.* **8**(4): 387–442.

Sheldon T (2004) Dutch reporting of euthanasia cases falls despite legal reporting requirements. *BMJ.* **328**: 1336.

Shue H (1996) *Basic Rights* (2e). Princeton University Press, New Jersey.

Slevin ML, Stubbs L, Plant HJ *et al.* (1990) Attitudes to chemotherapy: comparing views of patients wth cancer with those of doctors, nurses and general public. *BMJ.* **300**: 1458–60.

Smart JJC and Williams B (1973) *Utilitarianism: for and against.* Cambridge University Press, Cambridge.

Spurgeon B (2004) France passes 'Right to die' law. *BMJ.* **329**: 1307.

Steinhauser KE, Christakis NA, Clipp EC *et al.* (2000) Factors considered important at the end of life by patients, family, physicians and other care providers. *JAMA.* **284**: 2476–82.

Stone P, Phillips C, Spruyt O *et al.* (1997) A comparison of the use of sedative in a hospital support team and in a hospice. *Pall Med.* **11**: 140–4.

Sykes NP and Thorns A (2003a) The use of opioids and sedatives at the end of life in palliative care. *Lancet Oncol.* **4**: 312–18.

Sykes NP and Thorns A (2003b) Sedative use in the last week of life and the implications for end of life decision-making. *Arch Intern Med.* **163**: 341–4.

Symonides J (2003) *Human Rights: international protection, monitoring, enforcement.* UNESCO, Paris.

Thorns A (1998) A review of the doctrine of double effect. *Eur J Pall Care.* **5**(4): 117–20.

Thorns A and Sykes N (2000) Opioid use in the last week of life and implications for end of life decision-making. *Lancet* **356**: 398–9.

Tschann JM, Kaufman SR and Micco GP (2003) Family involvement in end of life hospital care. *J Am Geriat Soc.* **51**(6): 835–40.

Vlastos G (ed.) (1980) *The Philosophy of Socrates: a collection of critical essays.* University of Notre Dame Press, Indiana.

Webb P (ed.) (2005) *Ethics in Palliative Care* (2e). Radcliffe Publishing, Oxford.

White M (1997) *Isaac Newton: the last sorcerer.* Fourth Estate, London.

WHO (1990) *Cancer Pain Relief and Palliative Care* (Technical Report Series 804). WHO, Geneva.

Worthington R (2002) *Finding the Hidden Self.* Himalayan Institute Press, Philadelphia.

Yu J (2003) *The Structure of Being in Aristotle's Metaphysics.* Kluwer Academic Publishers, Dordrecht.

Further reading

British Medical Association (2004) *Medical Ethics Today.* BMA, London.

Campbell A, Gillett G and Jones G (2001) *Medical Ethics* (3e). Oxford University Press, Oxford.

Cooper DE (ed.) (1998) *Ethics: the classic readings.* Blackwell Publishing, Oxford.

Frey RG and Wellman CH (2003) *A Companion to Applied Ethics.* Blackwell Publishing, Oxford.

Garrett TM, Baillie HW and Garret RM (2001) *Health Care Ethics: principles and problems.* Prentice-Hall, New Jersey.

Glover J (1996) *Causing Death and Saving Lives.* Penguin Books, Harmondsworth.

Guyer P (ed.) (1998) *Kant's Groundwork of the Metaphysics of Morals: critical essays.* Roman and Littlefield, Oxford.

Hope T, Savulescu J and Hendrick J (2003) *Medical Ethics and Law: the core curriculum.* Elsevier Science, London.

Jonsen AR, Siegler M and Winslade WJ (2002) *Clinical Ethics: a practical approach to ethical decision in clinical medicine* (5e). McGraw-Hill, New York.

Loux ML (2002) *Metaphysics: a contemporary introduction* (2e). Routledge, London.

Machlin V (2003) *Medicolegal Pocketbook.* Churchill Livingstone, Edinburgh.

Mappes TA and Degrazia D (2001) *Biomedial Ethics* (5e). McGraw-Hill, New York.

Mason JK, McCall Smith A and Laurie GT (2002) *Law and Medical Ethics* (6e). Butterworths, London.

Montgomery J (2003) *Health Care Law* (2e). Oxford University Press, Oxford.

Schwartz L, Preece PE and Hendry RA (2002) *Medical Ethics: a case-based approach.* Elsevier Science, London.

Singer P (1996) *Rethinking Life and Death.* Palgrave Macmillan, Basingstoke.

Index

notes are denoted by n. following page numbers

Music Technology and Education

Music Technology and Education lays out the principles of music technology and how they can be used to enhance musical teaching and learning in primary and secondary education. Previously published as *Computers in Music Education*, this second edition has been streamlined to focus on the needs of today's music education student. It has been completely updated to reflect mobile technologies, social networks, rich media environments, and other technological advances. Topics include:

- Basic audio concepts and recording techniques
- Enhanced music instruction with interactive systems, web-based media platforms, social networking, and musicianship software
- Administration and management of technology resources
- Distance education and flexible learning

Music Technology and Education provides a strong theoretical and philosophical framework for examining the use of technology in music education while outlining the tools and techniques for implementation in the classroom. Reflective Questions, Teaching Tips, and Suggested Tasks link technology with effective teaching practice. The companion website provides resources for deeper investigation into the topics covered in each chapter, and includes an annotated bibliography, website links, tutorials, and model projects.

Andrew R. Brown is Professor of Digital Arts at Griffith University in Brisbane, Australia.